The Complicated Cataract

The Massachusetts Eye and Ear Infirmary Phacoemulsification Practice Handbook

Roberto Pineda II, MD
Massachusetts Eye and Ear Infirmary
Brigham and Womens Hospital
Boston, Massachusetts

Alejandro Espaillat, MD
Espaillat Cabral Eye Institute
Santo Domingo, Dominican Republic

Victor L. Perez, MD
Massachusetts Eye and Ear Infirmary
Boston, Massachusetts

Susannah G. Rowe, MD, MPH
Harvard Medical School
Boston University School of Medicine
Boston, Massachusetts

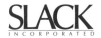

SLACK
INCORPORATED

an innovative information, education, and management company

6900 Grove Road • Thorofare, NJ 08086

Publisher: John H. Bond
Editorial Director: Amy E. Drummond
Design Editor: Lauren Biddle Plummer

The procedures and practices described in this book should be implemented in a manner consistent with the professional standards set for the circumstances that apply in each specific situation. Every effort has been made to confirm the accuracy of the information presented and to correctly relate generally accepted practices. The author, editor, and publisher cannot accept responsibility for errors or exclusions or for the outcome of the application of the material presented herein. There is no expressed or implied warranty of this book or information imparted by it. Any review or mention of specific companies or products is not intended as an endorsement by the author or the publisher.

The work SLACK publishes is peer reviewed. Prior to publication, recognized leaders in the field, educators, and clinicians provide important feedback on the concepts and content that we publish. We welcome feedback on this work.

The complicated cataract : the Massachusetts Eye and Ear infirmary phacoemulsification practice handbook / [edited by] Roberto Pineda... [et al.].
   p. ; cm.
   Includes bibliographical references and index.
   ISBN 1-55642-486-8 (alk. paper)
   1. Phacoemulsification--Handbooks, manuals, etc. 2. Cataract--Surgery--Handbooks, manuals etc. I. Pineda, Roberto. II. Massachusetts Eye and Ear Infirmary.
   {DNLM: 1. Cataract Extraction--Handbooks. WW 39 C7378 2001}
   RE451 .C65 2001
   617.7'42059--dc21   2001020081

Printed in the United States of America

Published by: SLACK Incorporated
         6900 Grove Road
         Thorofare, NJ 08086 USA
         Telephone: 856-848-1000
         Fax: 856-853-5991
         www.slackbooks.com

DEDICATION

To the people in my life who have unselfishly supported me through their generosity, kindness, and strength. And to Susannah, my ethereal enchantress, who has taught me the joy of sharing a life together.

Roberto Pineda, MD

I would like to dedicate my contribution to this book to my wife, Rosanna, and our wonderful daughter, Veronica Isabel. My deepest thanks to my colleagues Victor, Susannah, and in particular Roberto, for always believing in our efforts, and to John and Vikki at SLACK Incorporated for supporting our ideas.

Alejandro Espaillat, MD

To my beloved Odile Marie, for all the love and support she has always provided me with; and to our Victor Felipe, whose new, innocent laugh daily fills our lives with joy and energy for the future.

Victor L. Perez, MD

To my best friend and sweetheart Roberto, who brings me joy, and offers his wisdom with boundless generosity; and to our friends and family who encircle us with love and laughter.

Susannah Rowe, MD, MPH

CONTENTS

ACKNOWLEDGMENTS

We gratefully recognize the faculty, staff, and our colleagues at the Massachusetts Eye & Ear Infirmary for their instruction, guidance, and support of this project at all points along its completion. We owe a special debt of gratitude to both Dr. Magda Krzystolik for her support, critiques, and invaluable objective input during the preparation of this book, and J. D. Cavallerano, OD, PhD, for manuscript preparation and editorial assistance for Chapter 13.

Additionally, we wish to acknowledge Eric J. Arias and Edy G. Arias for their expert collaboration in preparing all the illustrations published in the book, without which this book would not be possible.

Finally, we thank our families for their encouragement, love, and support during the writing of this book, and Mary Rowe and Robert Fein for their gastronomic support during our long days and late nights.

Contributing Authors

Lloyd M. Aiello, MD
Joslin Diabetes Center
Harvard Medical School
Boston, Massachusetts

Robert T. Ang, MD
Massachusetts Eye and Ear Infirmary
Boston, Massachusetts

Theresa C. Chen, MD
Massachusetts Eye and Ear Infirmary
Boston, Massachusetts

Sandra L. Cramer, MD
Massachusetts Eye and Ear Infirmary
Boston, Massachusetts

C. Stephen Foster, MD, FACS
Massachusetts Eye and Ear Infirmary
Boston, Massachusetts

Melanie Kazlas, MD
Boston University School of Medicine
Boston, Massachusetts

Eugene S. Lit, MD
Massachusetts Eye and Ear Infirmary
Boston, Massachusetts

Richard J. Maw, MD
Massachusetts Eye and Ear Infirmary
Boston, Massachusetts

Sabera Shah, MD
Joslin Diabetes Center
Harvard Medical SchoolBoston,
Massachusetts

Christopher Starr, MD
Massachusetts Eye and Ear Infirmary
Boston, Massachusetts

Kailenn Tsao, MD
Massachusetts Eye and Ear Infirmary
Boston, Massachusetts

PREFACE

In our first editorial meeting, we agreed that the guidance of an experienced phaco surgeon represented one of the most important ingredients in learning phacoemulsification. We also concluded that careful preparation was essential when approaching potentially complicated cases, and that the generous advice of our mentors regarding preoperative preparations and postoperative management was at least as influential on our outcomes as guidance during the surgery itself. In addition to basic surgical concepts, these experienced surgeons offered seasoned judgment and bountiful "pearls" on preparing for diversely challenging cataract cases.

With this book we hope to provide the cataract surgeon with a compilation of suggestions and considerations that we have found useful when preparing for difficult phacoemulsification cases. We recognize that there are many strategies for managing each scenario, and we believe no single approach works well for all patients or for all surgeons. It is therefore vital to tailor one's approach based on individual circumstances. While in some instances we recommend a particular method that works well in our hands, we have tried in most cases to present several alternatives for consideration.

The modified outline format of the book facilitates rapid referencing whenever a challenging case is anticipated. It is our goal that you will find the book useful in the office while evaluating a patient, as well as in the surgical suite prior to surgery. In some cases, more than one chapter may apply. To minimize cross-referencing and to provide the surgeon with all the information needed in each chapter, we repeated certain information in multiple chapters throughout the book.

Most chapters follow a similar format, as follows: A brief review describes the Clinical Settings where the complicated cataract may occur. The list of Risks and Complications is useful when considering whether phacoemulsification surgery is appropriate and aids in consenting patients for the procedure. Pertinent History and Clinical Evaluation suggest possible additions to the standard preoperative evaluation. The section on Strategies to Maximize Outcomes enumerates preoperative preparations that may be helpful. Perioperative Considerations and Maneuvers addresses medications, anesthesia, and all relevant surgical steps (surgical steps that do not require special attention are excluded). Black and white figures illustrate important concepts. Since the book is intended for the ophthalmic surgeon who has basic phacoemulsification skills, we do not cover information about routine surgical steps that require no unusual attention. Special Maneuvers refers to any specialized surgical techniques that might be useful. When to Consider an Alternative Procedure highlights circumstances in which the surgeon ought to contemplate a different or additional procedure, or possibly no procedure at all. Finally, the Key Points emphasize the salient features of each cataract scenario and can be used for rapid review.

The information in this book derives from the teachings of our mentors, recently reviewed evidence from currently available ophthalmic literature, and our personal experience. As a warning, the recommendations provided in this book are only a guideline based on our opinion, and should not be taken as dogma.

In summary, with this handbook we wish to share some of the benefits we enjoyed while working with many generous, experienced mentors. Their many suggestions helped us to refine our decision-making, judgment, and preparation for challenging cases; we hope that in a similar way this guide will offer you food for thought while preparing for your own advanced phacoemulsification cases.

Roberto Pineda II, MD
Alejandro Espaillat, MD
Victor L. Perez, MD
Susannah G. Rowe, MD, MPH

FOREWORD

In the late 1960s and early 1970s, Dr. Charles Kelman introduced phacoemulsification clinical ophthalmic and surgical care for the removal of cataracts. I remember a course that Dr. Kelman gave in the early 1970s when I was a resident at the Edward S. Harkness Eye Institute of the Columbia Presbyterian Medical Center. Our Chief of Service, Dr. Arthur Geard DeVoe, attended the course and came back with glowing reviews of its potential for the future. When I went to Manhattan Eye, Ear, and Throat Hospital, I was privileged to get to know Dr. Kelman personally and, like others, was amazed at the playfulness of his mind and his openness to innovation. Phacoemulsification has now become the benchmark for the removal of cataract, and has paved the ground for our modern-day intraocular lens technology, particularly posterior chamber lenses with or without fixation.

As with any new surgical advance, some surgeons can make the transition, while others find it difficult or impossible. There is an increment in surgical dexterity that is required to obtain optimal outcomes. This text will become a constant companion to trainees and surgeons who are learning the ropes of phacoemulsification, as well as learning how to manage the inevitable complications that may ensue. Cataract surgery, with the methodology of phacoemulsification, has probably become the most successful invasive human surgery in the history of medicine.

The *Massachusetts Eye and Ear Infirmary Phacoemulsification Practice Handbook* has been spearheaded by Drs. Roberto Pineda II, Alejandro Espaillat, Victor L. Perez, and Susannah G. Rowe. These individuals have had connections with the Massachusetts Eye and Ear Infirmary, either as part of their training or as faculty members. From their varying perspectives, including a deep knowledge of intraocular inflammation and epidemiological aspects, they have produced a solid, reliable, and highly practical text for advancing the quality of ocular surgical care.

Frederick A. Jakobiec, MD, DSc (Med.)
Henry Willard Williams Professor of Ophthalmology,
Professor of Pathology, and Chairman of Ophthalmology
Harvard Medical School
Cambridge, Mass

Chief of Ophthalmology
Massachusetts Eye and Ear Infirmary
Boston, Mass

When is Cataract Surgery Appropriate?

Susannah G. Rowe, MD, MPH

Modern cataract surgery is one of the most successful interventions in the history of medicine. There is arguably no other medical procedure that provides as much benefit as quickly, painlessly, and inexpensively as cataract surgery. Cataracts are one of the most important causes of reversible disability in the elderly.[1-3] By any measure of success, appropriate cataract surgery improves patients' quality of life, general function, safety, and satisfaction.[3-8]

The success rate for cataract surgery may be as high as 80% to 90% depending on the outcome measure used.[4,5] Some surgeons report even higher success rates. However, all cataract surgeons eventually encounter patients who have failed to benefit from cataract extraction, as well as those who have had worse outcomes after surgery. Everyone involved wishes to minimize these unfortunate occurrences.

Phacoemulsification of complicated cataracts carries a higher risk of poor outcomes. The risk to benefit ratio for cataract surgery changes for these patients. Given the greater chance of adverse outcomes, it becomes especially important to ensure that cataract surgery is appropriate for high-risk scenarios. Fortunately, new research provides valuable clues as to who is most likely to benefit from cataract extraction. Although poor outcomes after cataract surgery are often difficult to predict (such as endophthalmitis), recent studies have identified some reliable preoperative predictors of cataract surgery success.[4,5] While the remaining chapters in this book address how to maximize outcomes for high-risk patients, this chapter will help surgeons decide when complicated cataract surgery is appropriate.

IMPORTANT PREDICTORS OF POSTOPERATIVE OUTCOMES

Better Outcomes

1. Worse visual disability preoperatively (vision-related quality of life, see below)
2. Younger age
3. Posterior subcapsular cataract

Worse Outcomes

1. Less visual disability preoperatively
2. Diabetes (with or without diabetic retinopathy)
3. Macular degeneration
4. Other ocular comorbidities (ie, PXE)
5. Postoperative anisometropia

VISION-RELATED QUALITY OF LIFE

Prevailing wisdom is changing regarding when cataract surgery is appropriate. In the past, many patients expected to undergo surgery when their cataract became "ripe." This determination was usually made by the surgeon and was based on whether the patient's visual acuity was significantly affected by the cataract. Patients often went to their doctors "to discover" whether they needed surgery.

Many prominent ophthalmic surgeons now believe that the need for cataract surgery should be primarily determined by the patient rather than by the surgeon. This decision is increasingly based on the patient's own needs, preferences, and functional limitations, in conjunction with their physical findings.

Preoperative visual disability (ie, vision-related functional difficulties and vision-related quality of life) is emerging as one of the most important predictors of postoperative outcomes. This factor is such an important predictor of cataract surgery success that some prominent and successful surgeons have abandoned relying on preoperative vision tests and now use vision-related quality of life as the only determinant of the need for cataract surgery. These surgeons will only operate when the cataract interferes with the patient's ability to perform needed and desired activities, and there is a reasonable likelihood of visual improvement after cataract extraction.

There are several survey "instruments" available that formally assess vision-related quality of life for cataract patients. These include the NEI-VFQ (Visual Function Questionnaire available from the National Eye Institute, Bethesda, Md [www.NEI.NIH.gov]), the VF-14 (National Eye Institute, Bethesda, Md), and the Cat-Quest.[9] These questionnaires take about 10 to 15 minutes to complete, and can be used to compare pre- and postoperative visual function.

An alternative to administering a formal questionnaire is to ask the patient relevant questions about his or her visual function. Some activities that are identified as important in quality of life studies are reading small print; reading traffic or street signs; doing fine handiwork or hobbies; cooking; driving (especially at night or under difficult conditions, like rain or traffic); walking down stairs, steps, or curbs (especially in dim light); recognizing faces and seeing people's expressions; and participating in sports.

OTHER COMMONLY ACCEPTED INDICATIONS FOR CATARACT SURGERY

While poor vision-related quality of life is the primary indication for cataract surgery, cataract removal is generally accepted under several other circumstances. These include lens-related complications, the need to visualize the fundus for diagnosis and/or treatment of other conditions (ie, glaucoma, macular degeneration, or diabetic retinopathy), children in the amblyopic age group with vision-obscuring cataract, and severe visual impairment in a patient who cannot communicate with the surgeon about difficulties related to vision. This indication is controversial, and probably should not be considered unless a close relative, guardian, or primary care physician is convinced that the patient has reduced quality of life related to the visual impairment.

DOCUMENTING INDICATIONS FOR SURGERY

It is important to document the need for surgery. This can be done in the clinic record or surgical dictation. Surgical dictations (operative reports) provide an opportunity to document the need for cataract surgery. This practice is useful for third-party payment and medical/legal reasons. Documentation need not be lengthy but should include the following elements: a description of the patient's visual symptoms, one or two examples of the patient's functional limitations, an assessment of whether the physical findings are consistent with the patient's complaints, an estimation of whether the surgery can be expected to yield visual improvement, confirmation that you have discussed the risks and benefits of the procedure with the patient, and reiteration of the patient's desire to proceed with the surgery.

The specifics will vary with individual circumstances. Below are sample dictations that we use in our clinical practice:

1. Mrs. Ramirez complains of increasing glare in the left eye, especially in bright light. Because of the glare, she sometimes has difficulty recognizing faces and avoids driving at night. Her symptoms are consistent with the posterior subcapsular cataract seen in her left eye. There is no evidence of other ocular conditions that may limit her visual function. I have discussed the risks and benefits of the procedure, and she desires cataract extraction for functional rehabilitation.

2. Mr. Jones has noticed progressive blurred vision in the left eye, which makes it difficult for him to walk without assistance. He has macular degeneration in the right eye, and a poor view of the fundus on the left eye due to 3+ nuclear sclerosis and 2+ cortical cataract. His visual symptoms are most likely due to macular degeneration as well as a cataract, given the status of the fellow eye. I have discussed the risks and benefits of surgery with him, including the limited prognosis for central vision after surgery. He wishes to proceed with surgery for functional rehabilitation of his peripheral vision.

3. Mr. Smith has early proliferative diabetic retinopathy and dense nuclear sclerosis in both eyes. His vision has remained stable at 20/400 OU and he has no visual complaints at this time. He has poor glycemic control and recent progression of the diabetic retinopathy. Since the cataract obscures adequate visualization of the fundus, I have recommended cataract surgery in the left eye to facilitate panretinal photocoagulation (PRP). I have discussed the risks and benefits of cataract surgery, including the possibility of progression of the diabetic retinopathy and the chance of no visual improvement, and the patient wishes to proceed with cataract extraction.

CONCLUSION

Indications for cataract surgery are changing, and greater patient participation is expected when determining the need for cataract extraction. Thoughtful discussion about the patient's visual limitations and vision-related quality of life is essential when preparing for cataract surgery. This is especially true when the risks from surgical complications and ocular comorbidity are higher. In the following chapters, we will discuss the possible risks and complications associated with each clinical scenario. This information, combined with an understanding of the patient's visual disability, will permit surgeons to maximize their chances of success and enhance patient satisfaction.

REFERENCES

1. Rahmani B, Tielsch JM, Katz J, et al. The cause-specific prevalence of visual impairment in an urban population. *Ophthalmology.* 1996;103:1721-1726.

2. Scott IU, Schein OD, West S, et al. Functional status and quality of life measurement among ophthalmic patients. *Arch Ophthalmol.* 1994;112:329-335.

3. Steinberg EP, Tielsch JM, Schein OD, et al. The VF-14: an index of functional impairment in patients with cataract. *Arch Ophthalmol.* 1994;112:630-638.

4. Mangione CM, Phillips RS, Lawrence MG, et al. Improved visual function and attenuation of declines in health-related quality of life after cataract extraction. *Arch Ophthalmol.* 1994;112:1419-1425.

5. Steinberg EP, Tielsch JM, Scein OD, et al. National Study of Cataract Surgery outcomes. Variations in 4-month postoperative outcomes as reflected in multiple outcome measures. *Ophthalmology.* 1994;101:1131-1141.

6. Brenner MH, Curbow B, Javitt JC, et al. Vision change and quality of life in the elderly. Response to cataract surgery and treatment of other chronic ocular conditions. *Arch Ophthalmol.* 1993;111:680-685.

7. Javitt JC, Brenner MH, Curbow B, et al. Outcomes of cataract surgery. Improvement in visual acuity and subjective visual function after surgery in the first, second, and both eyes. *Arch Ophthalmol.* 1993;111:686-691.

8. Rubin GS, Adamsons IA, Stark WJ. Comparison of acuity, contrast sensitivity, and disability glare before and after cataract surgery. *Arch Ophthalmol.* 1993;111:56-61.

9. Lundstrom M, Roos P, Jensen S, et al. Cat-Quest questionnaire for use in cataract surgery care: description, validity, and reliability. *J Cataract Refract Surg.* 1997;23(8):1226-1236.

THE COMPROMISED CORNEA

Susannah G. Rowe, MD, MPH
Roberto Pineda II, MD

RELEVANT PREOPERATIVE ISSUES

Clinical Settings

Cataract surgery in the presence of a compromised cornea presents unique challenges in both the perioperative and postoperative periods. Compromised corneas may limit visibility of the anterior chamber and lens, making ocular surgery more difficult. Compromised corneas may also exhibit increased vulnerability to the stress of phacoemulsification and may sometimes suffer prolonged inflammation with stromal thickening and endothelial decompensation, even after uncomplicated cataract extraction. In the setting of a compromised cornea, it is often advisable to modify one's phacoemulsification technique to maximize the postoperative outcome. The specific approach will depend in large part on the nature of the corneal pathology.

Clinically, it is useful to group corneal conditions into those diseases that primarily affect the epithelium, the stroma, or the endothelium.

Corneal Epithelial Diseases

Corneas with compromised epithelium can become rapidly cloudy during even short, atraumatic phacoemulsification and can severely limit the surgeon's view of the anterior chamber. Epithelial disease also can limit the eye's visual potential, depending upon its location and severity. Common relevant clinical settings are listed below:

- Diabetes mellitus
- Dry eye syndromes
- Rosacea
- Vernal keratoconjunctivitis (VKC)
- Cicatrizing conjunctivitis (eg, Stevens-Johnson syndrome)
- Exposure keratopathy (eg, lagophthalmos)
- Neurotrophic cornea (herpes simplex virus [HSV], and herpes zoster virus [HZV])

- Anterior corneal dystrophies of the epithelium and Bowman's layer
- Limbal stem cell deficiency states (eg, aniridia and chemical burns)

Corneal Stromal Diseases

Corneal stromal diseases can also limit visualization during phacoemulsification surgery due to focal or widespread stromal opacities. Usually the view remains stable throughout the surgery. Relevant conditions include:

- Arcus senilis
- Scarring (eg, previous corneal trauma or infections)
- Corneal degenerations (eg, keratoconus, pellucid marginal degeneration, Therrien's marginal degeneration)
- Incisional refractive surgery (eg, radial keratotomy and arcuate keratotomy)
- Interstitial keratitis (eg, herpes, syphilis, tuberculosis, or Lyme disease)
- Corneal stromal dystrophies
- Anterior crocodile shagreen
- Trachoma
- Other miscellaneous stromal opacities (eg, band keratopathy and Salzmann's nodules)

Corneal Endothelial Conditions

Corneal endothelial conditions can contribute to intraoperative corneal edema with decreased visualization. These conditions are also major contributors to postoperative corneal edema and prolonged visual rehabilitation:

- Fuchs' corneal endothelial dystrophy
- HSV/HZV
- Posterior polymorphous dystrophy (PPMD)
- Penetrating keratoplasty (PKP)
- Anterior uveitis
- Previous intraocular surgery
- Posterior crocodile shagreen

Risks and Complications

Patients with compromised corneas may have greater incidences of the following complications:

1. Reactivation of pre-existing herpetic eye disease
2. Prolonged corneal edema and haze
3. Irreversible visually significant corneal decompensation requiring penetrating keratoplasty
4. Transient hyperopic shifts in patients who have had radial keratotomy prior to cataract surgery
5. Rejection of corneal allograft in previous penetrating keratoplasty
6. Toxic damage to the corneal endothelium (eg, lidocaine and vancomycin)

7. Toxic epitheliopathy (eg, multiple topical medictations)
8. Intraoperative capsular complications due to poor visualization
9. Steroid-response glaucoma due to extended steroid use

Pertinent History

In addition to the usual ophthalmic history, surgeons should pay particular attention to the following:

1. History of previous ocular trauma, surgery, inflammatory disease, diabetes, or herpetic eye disease
2. History of fluctuating vision, worse in mornings (eg, Fuchs')
3. Dry eye symptoms
4. History of glaucoma with dorzolamide treatment
5. History of corneal complications (eg, prolonged edema, or PKP) related to cataract surgery in the fellow eye

Clinical Evaluation

The preoperative evaluation should include a comprehensive eye examination, with consideration of the following points, depending on the specific pathology:

1. Evaluate eyelid position and adequacy of blink; identify modifiable eyelid pathology (eg, entropion, ectropion, or trichiasis). Evert upper eyelids, examine tarsal conjunctiva for scarring (eg, Arlt's line, trachoma) or symblepharon (eg, cicatrizing conjunctivitis).
2. Assess meibomian gland function: look for inspissated, inflamed, or scarred meibomian glands (eg, meibomian gland dysfunction), erythema, swelling and telangectasias of eyelid margin (eg,rosacea), and small perilimbal corneal infiltrates near where the eyelid margins touch the cornea (eg,staph marginal disease).
3. Assess conjunctival goblet cell function: tear film break-up time (should be >10 seconds), presence of symblepharon, or other conjunctival scarring (eg, cicatrizing conjunctivitis).
4. Assess tear production: quantify basal tear secretion (use Zone Quick [Lacrimedics, Glendora, Calif] or Schirmer's test with topical anesthesia) and size of the tear lake (eg, keratoconjunctivitis sicca).
5. Assess corneal clarity: determine the quality of view into the anterior chamber, especially of the iris and anterior capsule.
6. Assess corneal and conjunctival epithelium with Rose Bengal (Akorn, Abita Springs, La) and fluorescein staining, look for staining patterns consistent with exposure (fine punctate staining of cornea and/or conjunctiva within the interpalpebral fissure), superior limbal keratitis (SLK) (dense Rose Bengal staining of superior limbus and bulbar conjunctiva). Identify corneal filaments, infiltrates, or other signs of active disease.
7. Consider corneal pachymetry to measure corneal thickness (if Fuchs' is suspected). Pachymetry is considered a better predictor of endothelial cell function than corneal endothelial cell counts. Patients with corneal thickness of >650

microns are more likely to need a penetrating keratoplasty after cataract surgery due to irreversible corneal decompensation.

8. Consider corneal endothelial cell count (eg,Fuchs'), and specular microscopy (especially for PPMD).

9. Evaluate depth of anterior chamber (to anticipate proximity of phacoemulsification probe to endothelium).

10. Evaluate density of the nucleus (eg,degree of nuclear sclerosis, brunescence, etc).

Strategies to Maximize Outcomes

1. To maximize patient satisfaction and promote realistic expectations, discuss any specific risks and complications of cataract surgery listed in the *Pertinent History* section that are relevant to your patient. Be sure to address possible limitations in visual acuity due to corneal opacities, as well as the possibility of prolonged corneal edema or irreversible corneal decompensation requiring penetrating keratoplasty.

2. Defer elective cataract surgery until all active corneal pathology (eg,corneal ulcers, herpetic dendrites, epithelial defects, or infiltrates) and uveitis are fully resolved for weeks to months.

3. For patients with herpetic corneal disease, the following should be considered:
   - It is preferable to delay elective cataract surgery until the cornea has been quiescent for at least 1 year (some authors state 6 months).
   - For recurrent herpetic epithelial and stromal disease.
     Consider pretreatment, starting the day before surgery, with antivirals (eg,acyclovir [400 mg po bid]) and/or topical antivirals, such as trifluridine 1% (eg,Viroptic [King Pharmaceuticals, Bristol, Tenn]) 9x/day, vidarabine 3% ointment (eg,Vira ATM [Monarch Pharmaceuticals, Bristol, Tenn]) 5x/day, or idoxuridine 0.1% (eg,Virex).
   - For herpetic disciform keratitis and herpetic immune endothelitis.
     Consider preoperative steroids (eg,prednisolone acetate 1% qid for 1 week prior to surgery).
   - While on topical steroids cover with topical antivirals (trifluridine 1% [eg,Viroptic] 5x/day, vidarabine 3% ointment [eg,Vira ATM] 3x/day, or idoxuridine 0.1% 3x/day [eg,Virex]).

4. Treat underlying eyelid pathology:
   - Baby shampoo lid scrubs, Blephamide (Allergan, Irvine, Calif) (for blepharitis and staph marginal)
   - Eyelash epilation (for trichiasis)
   - Warm compresses, doxycycline 50 mg po bid for 4 to 6 weeks (for rosacea or meibomian gland dysfunction)
   - Other eyelid procedures (for entropion, ectropion, and lid lag)

5. Treat dry eye signs and symptoms:
   - Use artificial tears. Consider silicone punctal plugs (eg, Oasis [Grafton Optical, Watford, UK] or EagleVision [Eaglevision, Memphis, Tenn] if dry eye findings are severe)

- Consider Theratears (Advanced Vision Research, Woburn, MA) for rapid tear film break-up time or history of goblet cell dysfunction (eg,cicatrizing conjunctivitis).

6. For patients with diabetes, consider pretreating with topical steroids (eg, prednisolone acetate 1%, one to two drops qid x 1 to 3 days) to minimize intraoperative and postoperative inflammation.

7. Consider pretreating patients who have loosely adherent corneal epithelium (eg, those with diabetes, recurrent erosions, corneal epithelial basement membrane dystrophy). Patients can be given ophthalmic sodium chloride 5% ointment the night before surgery, plus ophthalmic sodium chloride 5% solution upon awakening the day of surgery.

8. For patients with endothelial compromise who are using dorzolamide for intraocular pressure control, consider changing glaucoma medications prior to surgery. Dorzolamide has been associated with case reports of irreversible corneal edema after cataract surgery in some patients with compromised corneal endothelium.

PERIOPERATIVE CONSIDERATIONS AND TECHNIQUES

Immediate Preoperative Medications

1. Apply nonsteroidal anti-inflammatory (NSAID) medications and prednisolone acetate (one to two drops every 5 min x 3).

2. Maximize preoperative pupillary dilation in order to maximize the red reflex, with the following medications every 10 minutes x 3, starting 1 hour prior to surgery:
   - Phenylephrine 2.5% to 10%
   - Tropicamide 1%
   - Cyclopentolate 0.5% to 1%
   - Flurbiprofen 0.03% or Ketorolac tromethamine 0.5%[2]

Anesthesia Considerations

We recommend local anesthesia in compromised cornea cases. Avoid topical or intracameral anesthesia for patients with corneal endothelial compromise, as intracameral anesthesia has been shown to cause endothelial cytoplasmic swelling.[1]

Wound Construction

1. If an asymmetric corneal opacity is present, position the incision to maximize visualization of the anterior chamber (eg, temporal versus superior approach).

2. Avoid a long or tight corneal or scleral tunnel, which may compress the phacoemulsification probe sleeve and occlude flow of cooling solution, thereby leading to thermal tissue damage.

3. Consider a scleral tunnel rather than a clear corneal incision, especially in the setting of corneal endothelial disease or limbal inflammatory disease (eg, peripheral ulcerative keratitis/rheumatoid arthritis).

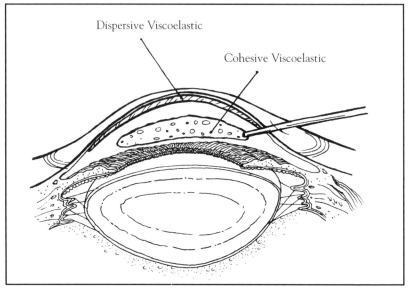

Figure 2-1. Employing the "soft shell technique", a dispersive viscoelastic is first used to coat the corneal endothelium, followed by a cohesive viscoelastic to maintain the anterior chamber.

4. Consider a clear corneal rather than scleral tunnel incision in the presence of conjunctival or ocular surface disease.

Viscoelastics Considerations

1. Use generous amounts of a viscodispersive viscoelastic with high coatability (<1 million Daltons, [eg, Viscoat]) to protect the corneal endothelium from mechanical trauma and to absorb phacoemulsification energy (Figure 2-1).

2. Consider the "soft shell viscoelastic technique" as described by Dr. S. Arshinoff, for patients with a compromised corneal endothelium. First inject a small amount of viscodispersive viscoelastic to coat the endothelium. Then inject a second, high molecular weight, highly cohesive viscoelastic (eg, ProVisc [Alcon, Fort Worth, Tex], Healon [Pharmacia & Upjohn, Bridgewater, NJ], Healon GV [Pharmacia & Upjohn, Bridgewater, NJ], or Amvisc Plus [Bausch & Lomb, Rochester, NY]) just above the lens capsule to absorb phaco energy. The second viscoelastic will push the first viscoelastic against the endothelium, creating a protective "shell" (hence the name).

Pupillary Considerations

Maximize dilation with topical mydriatics to enhance the view of the anterior capsule, lens, and red reflex in the setting of corneal opacity.

Capsulorrhexis and Other Capsular Considerations

1. For patients with an irregular corneal surface, try para-axial rather than coaxial illumination to improve the red reflex.

2. For patients with irregular corneal surfaces, consider placing a small amount of viscodispersive viscoelastic or artificial tears (eg, Ocucoat [Bausch & Lomb, Rochester, NY] or Celluvisc [Allergan, Irvine, Calif]) on the corneal epithelium to maintain visualization and to protect the loose epithelial layer.

3. Dimmed operating room lights, a good focus with high magnification, and frequent rewetting of the cornea are all helpful in successfully completing the capsulorrhexis.

Phacoemulsification

1. Be alert when introducing instruments to the eye, in order to avoid tears in Descemet's membrane.

2. Perform phacoemulsification in the pupillary plane to avoid insult to the corneal endothelium from excess energy.

3. Minimize contact between nuclear fragments and the cornea, since this trauma has been implicated as a primary cause of endothelial cell loss after cataract surgery.[2]

4. To lessen phaco energy transmitted to the corneal endothelium, a chopping technique is preferred over nuclear fractis (divide-and-conquer technique).

Cortical Aspiration

Careful cortical clean-up is necessary to reduce postoperative inflammation and resulting corneal endothelial cell damage.

Intraocular Lens (IOL) Implantation

1. Use adequate viscoelastic to protect the corneal endothelium during IOL implantation.

2. Ensure sufficient incision width for the implantation of the IOL to avoid excessive manipulation, force, or traction on Descemet's membrane.

3. We are unaware of any contraindications to any of the available IOL implant materials.

4. If a capsule-supported IOL is not possible, both sutured PCIOLs and open-loop ACIOLs have good corneal safety records.[3] The IOL choice should depend upon the surgeon's experience.

5. Measure corneal diameter and select appropriate ACIOL size carefully in order to avoid small loose ACIOLs, which may shift and cause increased intraocular inflammation and endothelial cell loss.

Special Techniques

1. In patients with high-risk corneal surface disease (eg, neurotrophic cornea, lagophthalmos), consider a temporary/partial tarsorrhaphy performed at the conclusion of surgery for added corneal protection.

2. An alternative to a tarsorrhaphy is a collagen corneal shield or bandage contact lens.

Immediate Perioperative Medications

1. Consider Diamox (acetazolamide) Sequels, 500 mg po bid to minimize postoperative corneal edema due to postoperative intraocular pressure (IOP) spikes.
2. Use a subconjunctival injection of dexamethasone immediately following cataract surgery to minimize postoperative inflammation.

RELEVANT POSTOPERATIVE ISSUES

Complications

1. Prolonged or permanent corneal edema. Patients with compromised corneas are at greater risk of irreversible corneal decompensation requiring penetrating keratoplasty after cataract surgery. The likelihood of corneal decompensation increases with the degree of corneal endothelial insult during surgery.
2. Recurrent herpetic disease.
3. Epitheliopathy. This can occur secondary to topical medications (especially NSAIDs and aminoglycosides) and exacerbated ocular surface disease.
4. Steroid-induced glaucoma.

Postoperative Medications

1. Consider intensive treatment with a topical steroid (ie, prednisolone acetate 1% one to two drops every 1 to 2 hours)
2. Consider NSAIDs (eg, ketorolac 0.5% [Acular] or diclofenac 0.1% [Voltaren]). However, use NSAIDs sparingly in the case of corneal epithelial compromise, since there have been reports of corneal epithelial toxicity with these medications.
3. Avoid aminoglycosides due to their potential for corneal epithelial toxicity.
4. Consider treating patients with recurrent severe ocular HSV infections with antivirals postoperatively: acyclovir (400 mg po bid for up to 18 months postoperatively) and/or topical antivirals (ie, trifluridine 1% [Viroptic] 9x/day or vidarabine 3% ointment [Vira ATM] 5x/day).
5. Treat IOPs above 21 mmHg for patients with any corneal endothelial compromise. Avoid dorzolamide due to its potential adverse effect on the corneal endothelium.
6. Aggressively treat patients with dry eye syndrome.

Follow-Up

1. More frequent follow-up visits should be considered if the patient has extensive corneal edema or intraocular inflammation, or if the patient has a history of herpetic eye disease.
2. If using high-dose steroids, more frequent visits are necessary to monitor IOP.
3. In patients with previous radial keratotomy, significant transient postoperative hyperopic shifts have been described. Delay any secondary procedures (eg, IOL exchange) until the refraction has stabilized (see Chapter 15).[4]

4. Consider placing collagen or silicone punctal plugs on the first postoperative day if signs of dry eye are severe.
5. Consider placing a bandage contact lens for corneal epithelial defects.

WHEN TO CONSIDER ALTERNATIVE PROCEDURES

1. In patients with evidence of clinical corneal edema, preoperative central corneal thickness of >650 microns by corneal pachymetry consider the need for combined cataract surgery and PKP.
2. In patients with active corneal disease, postpone surgery unless there is an emergency.
3. For compromised corneas with a suboptimal view of the anterior chamber, consider extracapsular cataract extraction (ECCE).
4. Consider an extracapsular surgical approach if the anterior chamber is very shallow, to preserve the corneal endothelium from trauma due to instruments, nuclear fragments, or very proximal phacoemulsification energy.
5. Consider an extracapsular surgical approach if the nucleus is very dense, to preserve the corneal endothelium from exposure to prolonged phacoemulsification energy and sharp nuclear fragments.

KEY POINTS

1. Avoid surgery until active corneal disease is stabilized.
2. Treat pre- and postoperative herpetic eye disease.
3. Avoid clear corneal incisions in patients with compromised endothelium.
4. Avoid scleral tunnel incisions in patients with ocular surface disease.
5. Consider phaco chop rather than the nuclear fractis technique in order to limit endothelial cell damage.
6. Use high-dose topical steroids liberally after surgery.
7. Consider tarsorrhaphy at the time of surgery in patients with neurotrophic corneas.
8. Monitor IOP and treat it aggressively in the presence of corneal endothelial compromise.

REFERENCES

1. Judge AJ, Najafi K, Lee DA, et al. Corneal endothelial toxicity of topical anesthesia. Ophthalmology. 1997;104(9):1373-1379.
2. Hayashi K, Hayashi H, Nakao F, et al. Risk factors for corneal endothelial injury during phacoemulsification. J Cataract Refract Surg. 1996;22(8):1079-1084.
3. Hardten DR. The cornea in cataract and intraocular lens surgery. Curr Opin Ophthalmol. 1996;7(1):43-48.
4. Koch DD, Liu JF, Hyde LL, et al. Refractive complications of cataract surgery after radial keratotomy. Am J Ophthalmology. 1989:108:676-682.

SUGGESTED READING

1. Sudaseh S, Laibson PR. The impact of the Herpetic Diseases Studies on the management of herpes simplex virus ocular infections. Curr Opin Ophthalmol. 1999;10:230-233.

3

THE SMALL PUPIL

Alejandro Espaillat, MD
Susannah G. Rowe, MD, MPH

RELEVANT PREOPERATIVE ISSUES

Clinical Settings

Small pupils (4 mm or less after dilation) occur in approximately 2% of patients. Small pupils are most commonly noted in the following conditions:[1]

- Advanced age
- Diabetes (iris ischemia ± rubeosis)
- Topical or systemic medications (miotics, narcotics)
- Pseudoexfoliation syndrome
- Uveitis (synechiae)
- Angle-closure glaucoma
- Trauma (synechiae)
- High hyperopia
- Neurological conditions (ie, Horner's syndrome)

Risks and Complications

Patients with a small pupil may have greater incidences of the following complications:

- Intraoperative and postoperative hyphema
- Postoperative inflammation from extensive iris manipulation
- Postoperative glaucoma from pigment, red blood cells (RBCs), or inflammation clogging the trabecular meshwork
- Iris trauma
- Temporary or permanent mydriasis with glare/diplopia
- Poor cosmesis, especially with light-colored irides due to irregular pupil
- Capsular tear (limited view of capsule and lens)

Pertinent History

In addition to the usual ophthalmic history, surgeons should pay particular attention to the following:

- History of complications (secondary to poor dilation) during cataract surgery in the fellow eye
- Glaucoma
- Uveitis
- Ocular and systemic medications (miotics, narcotics)
- Bleeding disorders
- Diabetes
- Trauma
- Hyperopia

Clinical Evaluation

The preoperative evaluation should include a comprehensive eye examination, with consideration of the following points, depending on the specific pathology:

- Observe pupil reactivity to light
- Measure pupil diameter after dilation
- Note presence of anterior or posterior synechiae
- Evaluate iris and pupil margin at slit lamp for evidence of rubeosis or signs of Fuchs' heterochromic iridocyclitis (gonioscopy may be indicated)
- Look for signs of pseudoexfoliation

STRATEGIES TO MAXIMIZE OUTCOMES

- To maximize patient satisfaction and promote realistic expectations, discuss any specific risks and complications of cataract surgery (including cosmetic issues) that are relevant to your patient.

- Maximize pupil dilation. Discontinue any miotic agent at least 3 days prior to surgery. Phosphylene iodide should be discontinued 3 weeks before surgery. Consider cyclopentolate 1% or scopolamine 0.25% one to two drops bid, 2 to 3 days prior to surgery.

- After consultation with the patient's internist, stop aspirin, oral NSAIDs and other anticoagulants (such as ginkgo biloba) 10 days prior to surgery due to risk of iris bleeding, particularly if extensive iris manipulation is anticipated.

- Controversy surrounds whether latanoprost is a risk factor for iris bleeding and cystoid macular edema (CME). We advise reviewing the ongoing literature and considering discontinuing latanoprost prior to surgery to minimize the risk of CME and iris bleeding.

- Consider preoperative topical steroids and topical nonsteroidal agents to minimize postoperative inflammation and risk of CME (see Appendix C).

- Lens choice should include an IOL with a 6.0 mm optic or larger to minimize optical aberrations in case the pupil is surgically enlarged. If excessive inflammation is anticipated, consider placement of a heparin-coated IOL (HSM CeeOn PMMA IOL [Pharmacia, Peaback, NJ]).

PERIOPERATIVE CONSIDERATIONS AND TECHNIQUES

Immediate Preoperative Medications

Maximize preoperative pupillary dilation with the following medications: Phenylephrine 2.5% to 10%, tropicamide 1%, cyclopentolate 0.5% to 1%, and flurbiprofen 0.03% or ketorolac tromethamine 0.5%. Drops should be given every 10 minutes x 3, starting 1 hour prior to surgery.[2]

Anesthesia Considerations

We recommend local anesthesia in these cases. Topical/intracameral anesthesia is not recommended due to anticipated uveal tissue manipulation. When administering retrobulbar or peribulbar anesthesia, beware patients who did not discontinue anticoagulants or who have bleeding disorders.

Wound Construction

Consider a scleral tunnel/limbal approach if there is an increased likelihood of conversion to an extracapsular procedure.

Viscoelastic Considerations

Choose a high molecular weight viscoelastic (eg, ProVisc, Healon, Healon GV, or Amvisc Plus) to aid in pupillary dilation, synechialysis, and hemostasis.

Pupillary Considerations

Surgeons should have a low threshold for surgically enlarging the pupil prior to the capsulorrhexis, especially if the pupillary diameter is no greater than 4.0 mm after maximal pharmacological treatment and generous use of a high molecular weight viscoelastic agent. This is important because poor visualization leads to a higher risk of serious intraoperative surgical complications. The following surgical techniques can be considered.

Synechialysis

- Viscosynechialysis: This maneuver should be attempted as a first-line treatment if iris adhesions are present. It is important to lyse all synechiae prior to stretching the pupil. Carefully separate the iris from the lens using the viscoelastic cannula and generous amounts of high molecular weight viscoelastic agents to allow a gentle and gradual pupillary dilation.

- In conjunction with viscoelastic, a Sinskey hook, Kuglen hook, or cyclodialysis spatula may be employed to release persistent synechiae.

Pupillary Stretching

- Pupil Stretch with two instruments: This is a popular and effective technique to enlarge a small pupil when mydriatic medications and viscoelastic agents are insufficient. It should be performed after viscoelastic is instilled into the anterior chamber, and the posterior synechiae are lysed. Two Graether collar buttons, a Kuglen hook and a Y-hook, or similar instruments can be used to mechanically stretch the pupil in the following manner. The two instruments are inserted into the anterior chamber. One button, or the Y-hook, engages the inferior pupillary margin while the other button, or Kuglen hook, engages the superior pupillary margin 180 degrees across from the first. The instruments are then gently and slowly moved simultaneously in opposite directions toward the iris root, and the stretch is maintained for 3 to 5 seconds. It is very important to stretch as far as possible into the angle, and to stretch very slowly to minimize iris trauma. Viscoelastic is then reinjected into the anterior chamber and the pupillary dilation is reassessed. If the pupil is still not adequately dilated, one can repeat the procedure 90 degrees from the first. If the second stretch is unsuccessful, one should attempt a different procedure (Figures 3-1 to 3-3).

- Pupil stretch with the Beehler pupil dilator: Four-point pupillary dilation is initiated by engaging the 12 o'clock pupillary margin with the primary microhook. During slow, controlled extension of the three other microfingers, all four hooks are engaged with the pupillary margin and gradually extended, resulting in a four-point symmetrical and simultaneous dilation of the pupil. The pupillary stretch is held at maximal dilation for several seconds, the hooks are slowly retracted, and the instrument is removed, leaving a dilated pupil. Another pupillary stretching device is the Peters pupil dilator (Rhein Medical Inc, Tampa, Fla) with an advancing loop and hook that expands to dilate the small pupil (Figure 3-4).

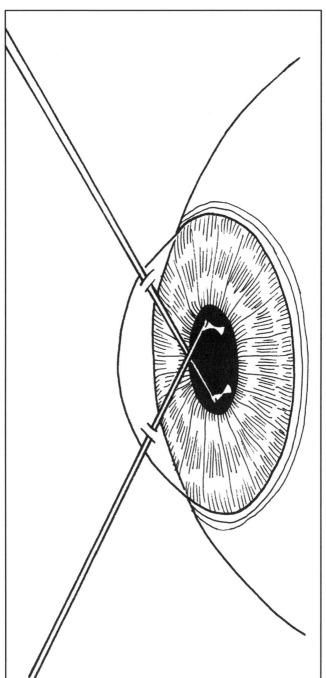

Figure 3-1. Pupil stretching technique using two instruments.

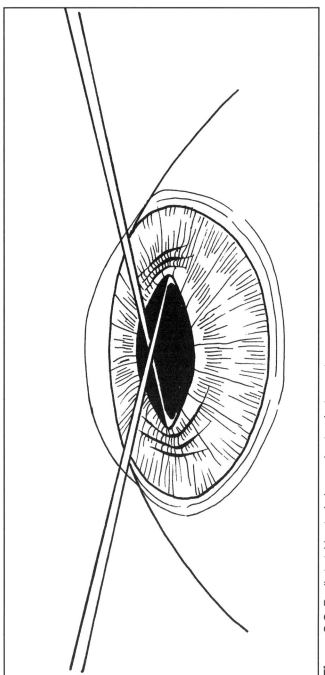

Figure 3-2. Pupil stretching technique using two instruments.

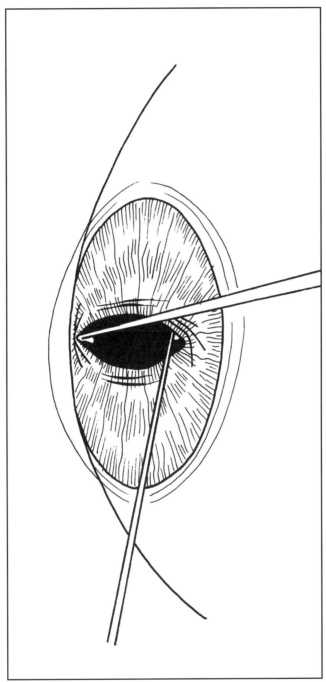

Figure 3-3. Pupil stretching technique using two instruments.

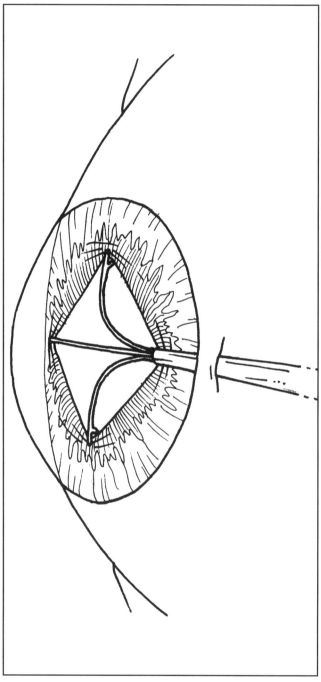

Figure 3-4. Pupil stretching technique using the Beehler pupil dilator.

Iris Retractors

- Nylon iris retractor hooks:[4] Flexible nylon iris retractors equipped with adjustable silicone sleeves are another option in pupillary dilation. Four equidistant paracentesis sites are made in the cornea, close to the limbus. It is very important to orient the incisions as peripherally as possible and flat to the iris plane, to prevent tenting of the iris margin after hook placement. The iris hook retractor is then inserted via the paracentesis incision to engage the pupillary margin. The hook is gently retracted to achieve the desired amount of pupil dilation. The external silicone sleeve is then slid forward to anchor the hook. The second retractor is placed 180 degrees from the first, followed in a similar manner by the remaining two. The iris retractors may be removed at any point during the phacoemulsification procedure if desired. Following the surgical procedure, the retractors are removed from the eye (Figures 3-5 and 3-6).

- Mackool self-retaining titanium mechanical hooks:[5] This technique involves four peripheral corneal hooks that are inserted through self-sealing limbal incisions of about 1.5 mm. A second instrument is used to stretch the pupillary margin peripherally until it engages the hooks. Following the surgical procedure, the retractors are removed from the eye (Figures 3-7 to 3-9).

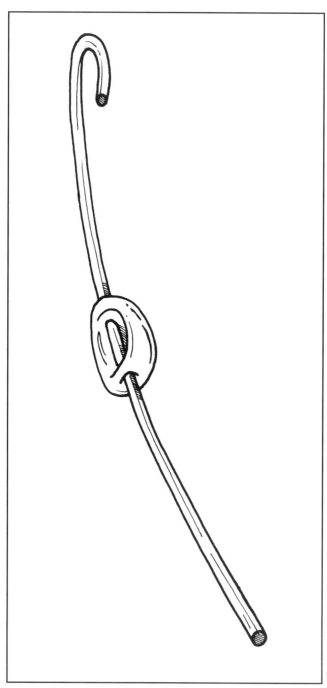

Figure 3-5. Pupil stretching technique using flexible nylon iris retractors equipped with adjustable silicone sleeves.

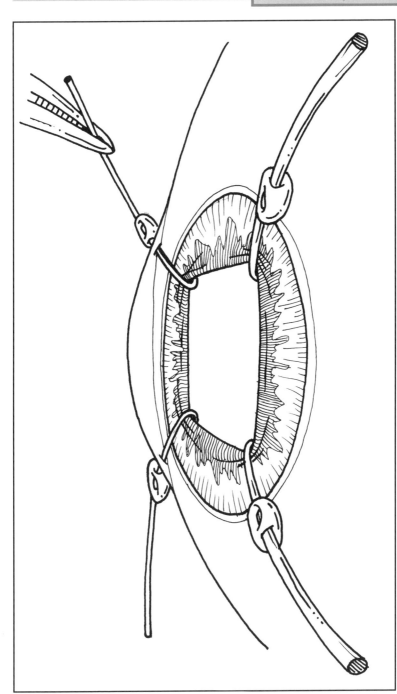

Figure 3-6. Pupil stretching technique using flexible nylon iris retractors equipped with adustable silicone sleeves.

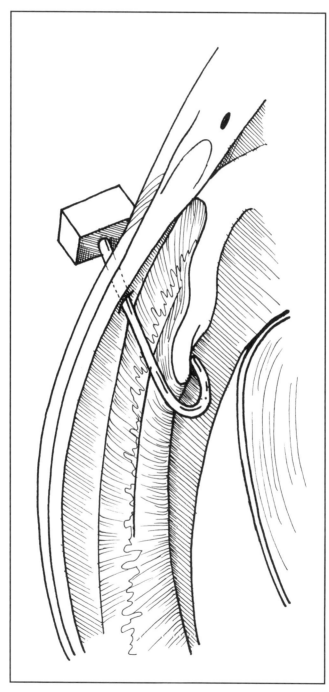

Figure 3-7. Pupil stretching technique using Mackool self-retaining titanium iris hooks and an iris pusher.

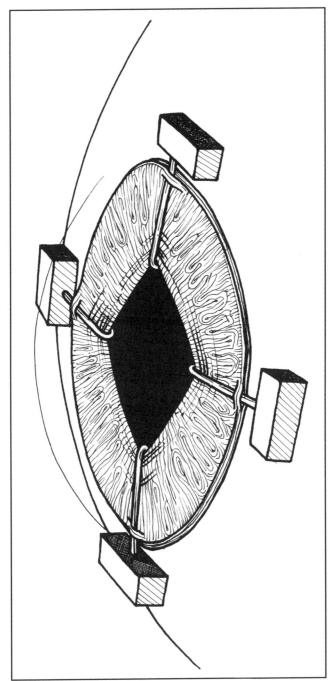

Figure 3-8. Pupil stretching technique using Mackool self-retaining titanium iris hooks and an iris pusher.

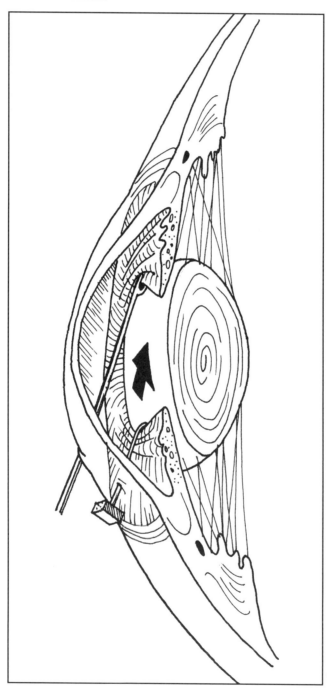

Figure 3-9. Pupil stretching technique using Mackool self-retaining titanium iris hooks and an iris pusher.

Graether Pupil Expander[6]

- The Graether pupil expander (EagleVision, Memphis, Tenn) uses a soft silicone ring with a circumferential groove, which engages the iris sphincter and allows sustained pupillary dilation during phacoemulsification and IOL implantation. The new 2000 version is preloaded and sterile, and features updates designed to improve ease of release and insertion (Figures 3-10 and 3-11).

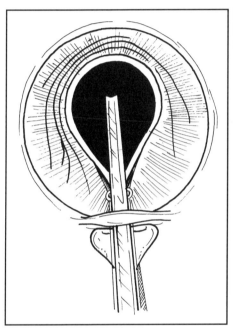

Figure 3-10. Pupil stretching technique using the Graether pupil expander's soft silicone ring.

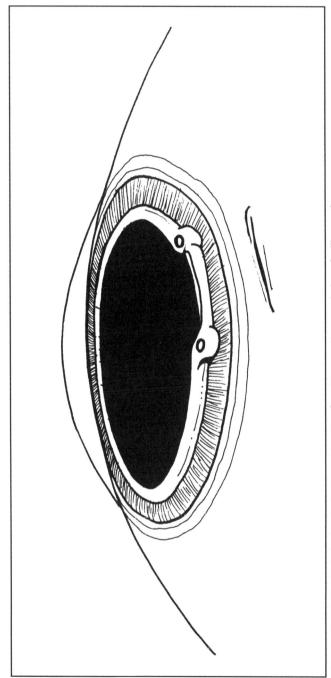

Figure 3-11. Pupil stretching technique using the Graether pupil expander's soft silicone ring.

Radial Iridotomy[7]

- This technique uses sharp scissors with long, fine blades. While angling the scissor blades horizontally to avoid damage to the anterior capsule, a long radial cut is made through the iris at 6 o'clock, resulting in a "key hole" pupil. Alternatively, the incision can be made at 12 o'clock by drawing the superior iris through the wound and creating a peripheral iridotomy. The peripheral iridotomy is then extended downward to the pupil via a radial cut with the scissors, taking care not to damage the anterior capsule. Because permanent optical alterations can result from sphincter damage, the defect is usually closed at the end of the procedure using a McCannel suture. Radial iridotomy can often lead to bleeding and increased inflammation; therefore, many surgeons do not consider it to be a first-line technique (Figures 3-12 and 3-13).

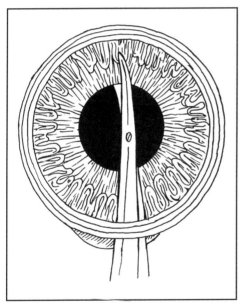

Figure 3-12. Pupil enlarging technique creating a radial iridotomy with long, sharp capsular scissors.

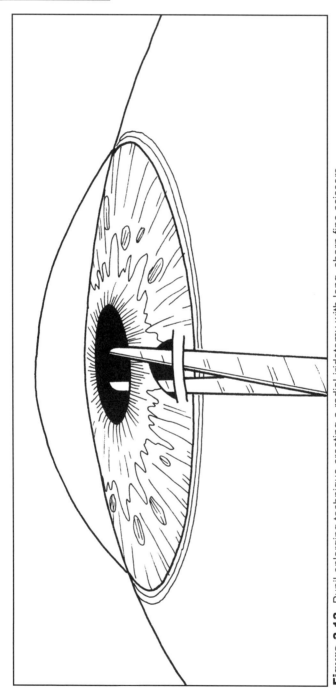

Figure 3-13. Pupil enlarging technique creating a radial iridotomy with long, sharp fine scissors.

Fine Incisional Pupilloplasty/Sphincterotomy[8]

- Using Rappazzo scissors, angled Gills or other long, fine scissors, eight microsphincterotomies (0.5 to 0.75 mm in length) are made at equal intervals about the pupillary border. The surgeon avoids cutting entirely through the sphincter and into the stroma. Viscoelastic agent is added to the anterior chamber for further dilation, usually achieving a diameter from 5.5 to 7 mm (Figures 3-14 and 3-15).

Capsulorrhexis and Other Capsular Considerations

Attempting a capsulorrhexis with a small pupil creates several difficulties: the red reflex is suboptimal, and either the capsulorrhexis is small or it must extend beneath the pupillary border. Neither situation is ideal, as a small capsulorrhexis leads to difficulty removing the nucleus, and it is potentially dangerous to perform the capsulorrhexis behind the iris due to poor visibility.

Because many surgeons consider the ideal capsulorrhexis diameter to be at least 5 mm, the pupil should be at least 5.0 mm before initiating the capsulorrhexis. If the pupil is less than 5.0 mm, additional pupil expanding techniques are probably necessary (as previously described). However, if the pupil is 6.0 mm or larger, a standard capsulorrhexis is usually feasible.

With a small pupil, it is important to have good control of the capsulorrhexis. Therefore, the technique should be performed slowly and with great care. Extra viscoelastic in the anterior chamber will help tamponade any iris bleeding, maximize visualization of the red reflex and capsular flap, and help prevent the capsulorrhexis from extending peripherally.

Hydrodissection

Thorough hydrodissection is essential to ensure easy nuclear manipulation and complete cortical removal when visualization is poor due to a small pupil. Use a 26-gauge blunt cannula to elevate the anterior capsular flap away from the cortical material. The cannula will maintain the anterior capsule in a tented-up position at the injection site. To ensure an effective fluid wave, it is important to insert the cannula far enough toward the equator to prevent reflux of fluid along the cannula barrel. Once the cannula is properly placed and the anterior capsule is elevated, continuous gentle irrigation will create the fluid wave and cleave the cortex from the posterior capsule in most locations. Repeating the hydrodissection in multiple quadrants is helpful. Make sure that the lens can spin freely within the capsular bag before proceeding with phacoemulsification.

Phacoemulsification

Any of the standard phacoemulsification[9,10] techniques can be used to remove the cataract. However, if the pupil remains small after pupil dilation, a nuclear chopping technique may be preferred over a nuclear fractis technique, depending upon lens density and capsular integrity. We recommend performing phacoemulsification in the pupillary plane, creating a deep central space, using low aspiration flow and a low vacuum rate to avoid inadvertent aspiration of the iris and posterior capsule.

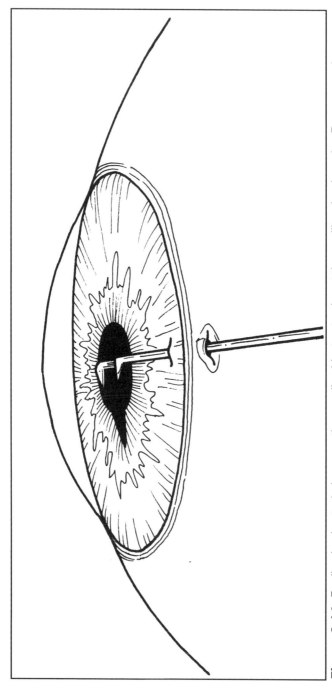

Figure 3-14. Pupil enlarging technique creating small sphincterotomies at the pupillary border using Rappazzo scissors.

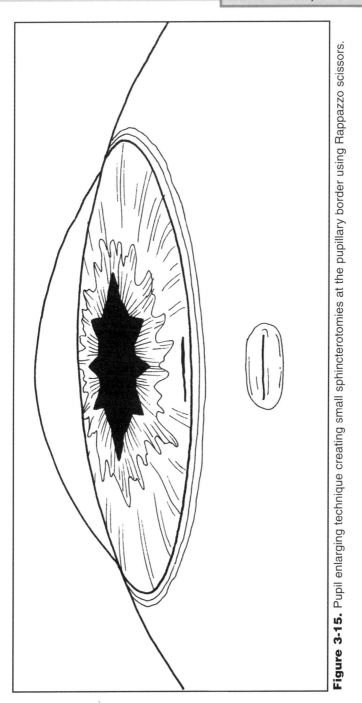

Figure 3-15. Pupil enlarging technique creating small sphincterotomies at the pupillary border using Rappazzo scissors.

Cortical Aspiration

Thorough cortical cleanup should be performed after phacoemulsification. A Kuglen hook or Y-hook can be used to retract the pupil, allowing direct visualization of any remaining cortical material.

IOL Implantation

Lens choice should include an IOL with a 6.0 mm or larger optic to minimize optical aberrations in cases where the pupil is surgically enlarged. Again, a Kuglen hook or Y-hook can be used to retract the pupil, allowing confirmation of the IOL position. If a larger capsulorrhexis is desired, it can be enlarged after insertion of the IOL and before aspiration of the viscoelastic. This is done using a cystotome to initiate a tear, which is then completed using the same instrument or the capsulorrhexis forceps.

Immediate Preoperative Medications

We recommend a subconjunctival injection of dexamethasone 20 to 40 mg immediately following cataract surgery to minimize postoperative inflammation.

Relevant Postoperative Issues

Complications

1. Cosmetic deformity of the iris (ie, mydriasis, irregular pupil).

2. Bleeding—usually self-limited and rarely requires treatment.

3. Inflammation—may be short-term or chronic. Consider intensive postoperative antiinflammatory treatment.

4. CME. Consider using both steroids and NSAIDs concurrently starting immediately after surgery (see CME algorithm in Appendix C).

5. Permanent optical aberrations and glare (mydriasis). Consider surgical repair if symptomatic.

6. Iris pigment dispersion (visually significant IOL deposits). Consider neodymium:yttrium-aluminum-garnet (Nd:YAG) laser optic dusting if the patient is symptomatic. When dusting, beware of silicone lenses, which can pit easily.

7. Postoperative glaucoma due to debris (blood, pigment, inflammatory cells) in the trabecular meshwork. May require glaucoma medications.

Postoperative Medications

1. Consider intensive treatment with a topical steroid (ie, prednisolone acetate 1% one to two drops every 1 to 2 hours) in case of extensive iris manipulation.

2. Consider NSAIDs, such as ketorolac 0.5% (ie, Acular [Allergan, Irvine, Calif] or diclofenac 0.1% (Voltaren [Novartis, East Hanover, NJ]).

Follow-Up

If significant iris trauma occurs during surgery or follow-up exams, be alert for signs of significant postoperative inflammation, elevated IOP, and CME. Consider more frequent postoperative visits to monitor these conditions.

WHEN TO CONSIDER ALTERNATIVE PROCEDURES

1. If pupil dilation techniques yield inadequate visualization, consider converting to an ECCE technique. Consider conversion particularly in cases of dense nuclear sclerosis and zonular instability (ie, pseudoexfoliation), where there is an increased risk of capsular disruption.

2. In advanced glaucoma cases, consider combined cataract and trabeculectomy.

3. If patients are on anticoagulants that cannot be discontinued safely, consider postponing the procedure due to the high risk of excessive iris bleeding and choroidal hemorrhage. Although anticoagulants are not considered an absolute contraindication, this surgery should be performed by a surgeon with extensive phacoemulsification experience due to the increased chance of long-term vision-threatening complications. For the beginning phacoemulsification surgeon, we do not recommend performing phacoemulsification surgery in patients with bleeding disorders and small pupils.

4. Avoid retrobulbar and peribulbar anesthesia for patients who cannot discontinue anticoagulants or who have bleeding disorders. Consider general anesthesia in these cases since topical anesthesia is a poor choice due to extensive iris manipulation.

KEY POINTS

1. Determine the cause of the small pupil.

2. Discontinue any miotic agent at least 3 days prior to surgery.

3. Treat any intraocular inflammation prior to surgery.

4. Consider starting nonsteroidal or steroidal topical medications 3 days before surgery.

5. Obtain maximal pharmacologic dilation prior to surgery.

6. Use high-molecular weight viscoelastic agents.

7. Have a low threshold to enlarge the pupil.

8. Use the least invasive technique that effectively dilates the pupil. We prefer any of the pupillary stretching techniques or mechanical iris dilators.

9. Perform a slow, well-controlled capsulorrhexis.

10. Assess potential for uncontrolled bleeding.

REFERENCES

1. Dinsmore SC. Modified stretch technique for small pupil phacoemulsification with topical anesthesia. *J Cataract Refract Surg.* 1996;22:27-30.

2. Solomon KD, Turkalj JW, Wjiteside SB, et al. Topical 0.5% Ketorolac vs. 0.03% Flubiprofen for inhibition of miosis during cataract surgery. *Arch Ophthalmol.* 1997;115:1119-1122.

3. Nelson DB, Donnenfeld ED. Small pupil phacoemulsification and trabeculectomy. *Int Ophthalmol Clin.* 1994;34:131-144.

4. Nichamin LD. Enlarging the pupil for cataract extraction using flexible nylon iris retractors. *J Cataract Refract Surg.* 1993;19:793-796.

5. Mackool RJ. Small pupil enlargement during cataract extraction. *J Cataract Refract Surg.* 1992;18:523-556.

6. Graether JM. Graether pupil expander for managing the small pupil during surgery. *J Cataract Refract Surg.* 1996;22:530-535.

7. Faust KJ. Modified radial iridotomy for small pupil phacoemulsification. *J Cataract Refract Surg.* 1991;17:866-867.

8. Fine IH. Pupilloplasty for small pupil phacoemulsification. *J Cataract Refract Surg.* 1994;20:192-196.

9. Koch PS. Small pupil phacoemulsification. In: Koch PS. *Simplifying Phacoemulsification: Safe and Efficient Methods for Cataract Surgery.* 5th ed. Thorofare, NJ: SLACK Incorporated; 1997.

10. Vasavada A, Singh R. Phacoemulsification in eyes with a small pupil. *J Cataract Refract Surg.* 2000;26:1210-1218.

4

PSEUDOEXFOLIATION SYNDROME

Robert T. Ang, MD
Susannah G. Rowe, MD, MPH
Roberto Pineda II, MD

RELEVANT PREOPERATIVE ISSUES

Clinical Settings

The prevalence of pseudoexfoliation syndrome (PXF) has been reported to range from as low as 0.2% (Japan) to as high as 20% (Finland),[1] and is seen most commonly among people of Scandinavian descent. The condition is uncommon in people younger than 50 years of age, but the incidence nearly doubles every decade thereafter.[2] From 48% to 76% of cases appear to be unilateral at diagnosis, according to reports. At diagnosis, one-fifth of patients with PXF are also found to have concomitant glaucoma or elevated IOP. Those with normal IOP and no glaucoma at diagnosis have a 5% chance of acquiring an elevated IOP within 5 years, and a 15% chance of developing elevated IOP within 10 years.[1]

Risks and Complications

Patients with pseudoexfoliation syndrome may have greater incidences of the following complications:

1. Zonular breaks (2.6%),[3] zonulolysis (13.1% to 17.9%)[4]
2. Phacodonesis (8.4%)[4]
3. Subluxation of lens (10.6%)[4]
4. Capsular tear (2.1%)[3]
5. Vitreous loss (5 to 11%)[4]
6. Postoperative inflammation
7. Poor dilation
8. Pupillary block glaucoma
9. Secondary angle-closure glaucoma
10. Capsular contraction syndrome
11. CME (related to items 1 to 6 above)

Pertinent History

In addition to the usual ophthalmic history, surgeons should pay particular attention to the following:

1. History of glaucoma

2. Visual disturbance (such as unstable refraction due to lens subluxation)

3. History of complications during cataract surgery in the fellow eye

Clinical Evaluation

The preoperative evaluation should include a comprehensive eye examination, with consideration of the following points, depending on the specific pathology:

1. Dilate the pupil (as many as 20% of pseudoexfoliation cases will be missed if examined without dilation).[5] On dilated slit lamp examination, the hallmark sign is grey-white, with dandruff-like deposits and flakes on the anterior surface of the iris and pupillary margin. The deposits are scattered across the anterior surface of the crystalline lens, except for a doughnut-shaped clear ring just behind the pupillary margin.

2. Dilated slit lamp examination is the best method for detecting subtle signs of zonular instability, including lens dislocation, iridodonesis, or phacodonesis. These findings can be elicited if the patient makes several rapid eye movements at the slit lamp. Older patients are more likely to have these findings.

3. It is strongly recommended that these patients undergo gonioscopy prior to cataract extraction. If the trabecular meshwork has become clogged with pseudoexfoliation debris and pigment, additional measures may be necessary to control the IOP.

4. It is well-recognized that patients with pseudoexfoliation do not dilate well. Therefore, measure the pupil size after maximal pharmacologic dilation to prepare for any necessary intraoperative dilation (see Chapter 3).

5. Perform a complete glaucoma evaluation, including assessment of the optic nerve, IOP, and visual field examination if necessary.

STRATEGIES TO MAXIMIZE OUTCOMES

1. To maximize patient satisfaction and promote realistic expectations, discuss any specific risks and complications of cataract surgery that are relevant to your patient. Focus on the risk of capsular rupture and its complications, including IOL placement issues.

2. Maximize pupil dilation. Discontinue any miotic agent at least 3 days prior to surgery. Pay special attention to phosphylene iodide, which should be discontinued 3 weeks before surgery. Consider cyclopentolate 1% or scopolamine 0.25% one to two drops bid, 2 to 3 days prior to surgery.

3. Optimize the management of any pre-existing glaucoma.

4. Use CME prophylaxis medications preoperatively (see Appendix C).

IOL Considerations

A 6.0-mm optic IOL allows an extra margin of safety if the IOL becomes mildly decentered. Ideally, the overall IOL diameter should be 13 mm and no smaller than 12.0. PMMA haptics are often preferred since they are stiffer and may help prevent capsular contraction and IOL decentration. We have used the following IOLs with good results: foldable one-piece acrylic, foldable acrylic with PMMA haptics, and one-piece PMMA.

PERIOPERATIVE CONSIDERATIONS AND TECHNIQUES

Immediate Preoperative Medications

Maximize preoperative pupillary dilation with the following medications: Phenylephrine 2.5% to 10%, tropicamide 1%, cyclopentolate 0.5% to 1%, and flurbiprofen 0.03% or ketorolac tromethamine 0.5% every 10 minutes x 3, starting 1 hour prior to surgery.

Anesthesia Considerations

Avoid stressing the zonules by overpressuring the eye. For this reason, it is best to avoid compression of the globe after applying anesthesia (ie, avoid digital massage, Super-Pinky [Hedstrom Toys, Bedford, Pa], or Honan balloon). For the same reason, do not inject an excessive volume of anesthesia during a peribulbar or retrobulbar injection.

Topical and intracameral anesthesia should be avoided in cases of phacodonesis and zonular dialysis.

Wound Construction

Consider a short scleral tunnel approach, which will facilitate conversion to ICCE or ECCE if needed. A relatively short, wider wound can lessen the risk of hyperinflation of the anterior chamber and resultant zonular traction from posterior displacement of the lens.

Viscoelastic Considerations

Use a high molecular weight, highly cohesive viscoelastic (eg, ProVisc, Healon, Healon GV, or Amvisc Plus) to facilitate dilation of the pupil and help control iris bleeding should pupil enlarging techniques be employed.

Avoid hyperinflation of the anterior chamber while injecting viscoelastic, as this can force the lens posteriorly and rupture the zonules.

Pupillary Considerations

A nondilating small pupil can be managed in a variety of ways: sector iridectomy, iris hooks such as the Kuglen and Y-hook, or pupil stretching with a Beehler pupil dilator, which stretches the pupil to 6.0 to 7.0 mm while creating tiny microsphincterotomies circumferentially around the pupil. Iris hooks and pupil retractors allow more controlled pupil dilation and, thus, less surgical trauma (see Chapter 3).

Capsulorrhexis and Other Capsular Considerations

The capsulorrhexis should be no smaller than 5 mm (ideally larger) to minimize the risk of postoperative capsular contraction.[6] The surface of the lens capsule can be hard to perforate with a cystotome without excessive downward force on the lens. Pinch-type forceps (ie, Kershner capsulorrhexis cystotome forceps [Rhein Medical, Tampa, Fla]) have sharp tips that simultaneously grasp the capsule and initiate the tear without pressing down onto the lens. Avoid excessive traction opposite the areas of zonular weakness. If it is difficult to complete a continuous curvilinear capsulorrhexis without stressing the zonules, consider converting to a beer can-style capsulotomy. Should radialization occur, have a low threshold to convert to ECCE.

Hydrodissection

Hydrodissection is extremely important in these cases, since it lessens traction on the zonules during rotation of the lens and during cortical aspiration. Gentle subcapsular hydrodissection should be carried out in multiple quadrants to thoroughly sever cortico-capsular adhesions until the lens rotates freely. Avoid overinflating the anterior chamber while performing hydrodissection, as this can push the lens-iris diaphragm posteriorly and challenge the zonules. Hyperinflation can be prevented by tilting the hydrodissection cannula slightly vertically or using it to depress the posterior lip of the wound gently, thus allowing the wound to leak slightly. Hydrodelineation is not recommended since it can produce a thicker cortical shell, which may stress zonules on removal.

Phacoemulsification

Minimize displacement of the lens while removing the nucleus. Standard divide-and-conquer techniques can stress the zonules; therefore, we suggest the use of a non-rotational cracking or chopping technique. Use sufficient power to minimize lens displacement, and consider a high-cavitation phaco tip (eg, a Kelman tip [Alcon, Fort Worth, Tex]) that emulsifies nuclear material beyond the tip and thereby minimizes dragging of the lens while sculpting. This technique allows an initial groove to be formed. Without rotating the lens, a lateral and rotational motion of the phaco probe can groove the nucleus in a lateral direction.[7]

Stabilize the nucleus with a second instrument through the paracentesis site if lens movement is noted during phacoemulsification. One can also push the nucleus toward the phaco tip while elevating the lens slightly. If rotation is necessary, do so using both instruments simultaneously placed at opposite poles of the nucleus to maximize spinning without stressing the zonules.

Keep the bottle height low to minimize hyperinflation of the anterior chamber and downward stress on the zonules.

Cortical Aspiration

If there is an area of suspected zonular instability, consider placing the IOL prior to cortical removal. Positioning one haptic at the point of zonular instability may help support the capsular bag and zonules in this area. Do not drag the cortex centrally; it is safer to strip it tangentially. Apply forces in the direction of any areas of zonular dehiscence rather than away from them. Injecting viscoelastic between the cortex and capsule (ie, viscodissection) sometimes aids in less traumatic cortex removal.

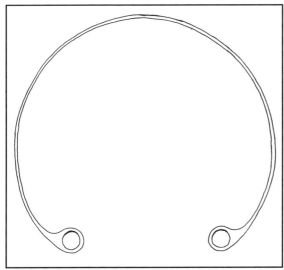

Figure 4-1. The Morcher endocapsular ring from Germany is made of PMMA and is available in three sizes: 10 mm (normal), 11 mm (large), and 12 mm (extra large). Larger sizes are designed for longer myopic eyes.

Keep the bottle height low to minimize hyperinflation of the anterior chamber and downward stress on the zonules.

Special Techniques

Capsular Ring

- An endocapsular ring is placed inside the capsular bag immediately after the capsulorrhexis to keep the bag stretched throughout the procedure.[7,8] The rings come in three sizes (normal = 10 mm, large = 11 mm, extra large = 12 mm). Endocapsular rings distribute any forces to the entire zonular ring, stabilizing the equator of the bag during cortical aspiration, and expanding the bag to facilitate IOL implantation. The ring remains in place after surgery and helps resist capsular contraction due to metaplasia and fibrosis (Figure 4-1).

Microhooks

- Capsular microhook retractors are similar to pupillary retractors. They can be used in conjunction with endocapsular rings or by themselves. Four small, flexible hooks are inserted through corneal paracentesis sites to capture the capsulorrhexis edge. The hooks are then retracted gently, stretching the capsulotomy and stabilizing the lens at four points.[8] The hooks lessen rotational as well as posterior movement of the bag. They are removed at the end of the case.

IOL Implantation

Verify that the capsular bag is intact and that there is sufficient zonular support for the bag prior to placing an endocapsular or sulcus-fixated IOL. If there is doubt as to sufficient zonular support (greater than 4 clock hours), consider an anterior chamber IOL.

When placing foldable IOLs, consider folding the lens in the "taco" configuration or using an injector such that both haptics will unfold simultaneously into the bag. This will lessen rotational traction on the zonules. Otherwise, consider "dunking" rather than rotating (dialing) the trailing haptic for the same reason.

If the capsular bag appears to be well-supported, but there is an area of suspected zonular instability, position one haptic at the point of weakness to help support the capsular bag and zonules in this area. This will also help prevent prolapse of vitreous anteriorly.

RELEVANT POSTOPERATIVE ISSUES

Complications

1. Postoperative iris deformity due to iris trauma, mechanical stretching, or sphincterotomy. Inadequate mydriasis was the major intraoperative difficulty observed in 48.4% of cases in one series.[9]

2. Increased postoperative inflammation has been correlated with inadequately dilated pupils,[10] possibly due to iris trauma with pigment release.

3. Postoperative capsule shrinkage and IOL decentration/tilt may result from unopposed capsular contraction in the setting of zonular weakness.[11]

4. IOL subluxation when zonular support is inadequate.

5. Posterior capsular opacification: an Nd:YAG laser anterior capsulotomy can be performed when the patient's vision is impaired by capsular fibrosis. Delay the procedure until 3 months after surgery due to increased risk of retinal detachment.

6. CME (see Appendix C).

Postoperative Medications

1. Treat with a topical steroid, NSAIDs (ie, ketorolac 0.5% [Acular] or diclofenac 0.1% [Voltaren]), and topical antibiotics.

2. If capsular rupture has occurred, refer to Appendix C for CME treatment options.

Follow-Up

1. More frequent follow-up visits should be considered if zonular tear, capsular break, or vitreous loss is encountered during surgery.

2. Anterior chamber inflammation and IOP should be well-controlled.

3. Perform an early dilated examination to assess IOL positioning and support if zonular instability is suspected.

WHEN TO CONSIDER ALTERNATIVE PROCEDURES

1. Inadequately controlled glaucoma. Consider phacoemulsification combined with a glaucoma procedure.[12]

2. Phacodonesis, iridodonesis, lens subluxation. Consider ICCE or ECCE.

3. Previous pars plana vitrectomy. Consider ECCE.

4. Advanced age (ie, >80 years old). Consider ECCE since the zonules are likely to be highly unstable by this age.

5. Dense nucleus. Consider ECCE.

KEY POINTS

1. Zonular breaks, capsular dialysis, or vitreous loss are 5 to 10 times more common in these cases, and may occur despite the most gentle and atraumatic surgery.

2. Begin prophylactic anti-inflammatory treatment for CME prior to surgery (see Appendix C).

3. Assess zonular integrity preoperatively.

4. Measure pupillary dilation. Perform surgical dilation if pharmacologic dilation is inadequate.

5. Optimize management of any glaucoma.

6. Avoid a Honan balloon, Super-Pinky, or digital massage.

7. Make the capsulorrhexis >5 mm if possible.[13]

8. Avoid hyperinflation of the anterior chamber.

9. Minimize displacement of the lens throughout surgery. Avoid tractional forces directed away from suspected zonular weak points.

10. Verify zonular stability prior to placing an IOL.

11. Perform early dilated examination to assess IOL positioning and support if zonular instability is suspected.

REFERENCES

1. Johnson DH. The exfoliation syndrome: a continuing challenge. In: Albert DM, Jakobiec EA, eds. *Principles & Practice of Ophthalmology*. 2nd ed. Philadelphia, Pa: WB Saunders Co. 1999:2718-2730.

2. Ekstom C. Prevalence of pseudoexfoliation in a population of 65-74 years of age. *Acta Ophthalmol*. 1987;65:9.

3. Scorolli L, Scorolli L, Campos E, et al. Pseudoexfoliation syndrome: a cohort study on intraoperative complications in cataract surgery. *Ophthalmologica*. 1998;212:278-80.

4. Kuchle M, Viestenz A, Martus P, et al. Anterior chamber depth and complications during cataract surgery in eyes with pseudoexfoliative syndrome. *Am J Ophthalmol*. 2000;129:281-85.

5. Forsius H. Exfoliation syndrome in various ethnic populations. *Acta Ophthalmol*. 1988;66:71.

6. Joo CK, Shin JA, Kim JH. Capsular opening contraction after continuous curvilinear capsulorrhexis and intraocular lens implantation. *J Cataract Refract Surg*. 1996;22:585-90.

7. Fine IH, Hoffman RS. Phacoemulsification in the presence of pseudoexfoliation: challenges and options. *J Cataract Refract Surg*. 1997;23:160-65.

8. Lee V, Bloom P. Microhook capsule stabilization for phacoemulsification in eyes with pseudoexfoliation-syndrome-induced lens stability. *J Cataract Refract Surg*. 1999;25:1567-70.

9. Alfaiate M, Leite E, Mira J, et al. Prevalence and surgical complications of pseudoexfoliation syndrome in Portuguese patients with senile cataract. *J Cataract Refract Surg*. 1996;22:972-76.

10. Drolsum L, Haaskjold E, Sandvig K. Phacoemulsification in eyes with pseudoexfoliation. *J Cataract Refract Surg*. 1998;24:787-91.

11. Hayashi H, Hayashi K, Nakao F, et al. Anterior capsule contraction with intraocular lens dislocation in eyes with pseudoexfoliation. *Br J Ophthalmol*. 1998;82:1429-1432.

12. Ritch R. Exfoliation syndrome. In: Ritch R, Shields MB, Krupin T, eds. *The Glaucomas*. 2nd ed. St. Louis, Mo: Mosby; 1996:993-1022.

13. Davidson JA. Capsule contraction syndrome. *J Cataract Refract Surg*. 1993;19:582-89.

5

THE UVEITIC EYE

Victor L. Perez, MD
C. Stephen Foster, MD, FACS

RELEVANT PREOPERATIVE ISSUES

Clinical Settings

Approximately 50% of patients who have different forms of uveitis eventually develop visually significant cataract.[1] The duration and location of the ocular inflammation, as well as the prolonged use of corticosteroids, are strongly related to the formation of cataracts with uveitis. Posterior subcapsular cataracts commonly result from the use of corticosteroids as well as from inflammation of the ciliary body.[2] Lens damage caused by the inflammatory response is thought to occur from a combination of mechanisms including free-radical production, deposition of immune complexes on the lens capsule, and the direct effect of proinflammatory cytokines such as interleukin-1 and tumor necrosis factor-alpha.[3-5] Anterior subcapsular changes also occur secondary to episodes of severe inflammation, which lead to posterior synechiae formation and areas of localized necrosis on the anterior capsular surface.

The visual outcome of patients with uveitis who undergo cataract surgery depends on the degree of trauma from the surgery itself, the amount of previous uveitic damage to essential ocular structures, and the degree and duration of postoperative inflammation. In a cohort study of patients with sarcoid uveitis who underwent cataract surgery, 61% achieved 20/40 vision postoperatively.[6] Damage from chronic posterior uveitis was the primary cause of postoperative vision worse than 20/40 in this population.[6] Other groups have made similar observations. In a study of 65 patients with VKH who underwent cataract surgery after control of the inflammation, 68% of the eyes had final visual acuity of 20/40 or better.[7] The most common reason for less than 20/20 vision was the presence of macular pathology. Heger et al[8] have also shown that 58% of uveitic patients undergoing cataract surgery with inflammation in remission achieved corrected visual acuity equivalent to 20/32. Posterior segment pathology was present in the eyes with poor outcome. Therefore, long-term control of intraocular inflammation in uveitic patients will not only help reduce the formation of cataract in these patients, but will maximize a good outcome when cataract surgery is needed by preventing ocular damage to vital structures in the eye pre- and postoperatively.

There are four types of uveitic patients who are likely to benefit from cataract extraction: those with uveitis caused by lens protein leakage (ie, phacoantigenic uveitis), those with a visually significant cataract when inflammation has been under long-term control, those whose cataract impairs visualization of the posterior segment for evaluation and follow-up of uveitis, and those whose cataract impairs necessary posterior segment surgery or other treatments.[2] Proper understanding of the medical management of patients with uveitis is essential for a successful outcome after cataract surgery.

Risks and Complications

Patients with uveitis may have greater incidences of the following complications:

1. Uncontrolled postoperative inflammation.

2. Corneal edema (see Chapter 2).

3. Posterior synechiae/pupillary sclerosis/membrane formation: these can limit surgical access to the lens because of poor pupil dilation (see Chapter 3).

4. Iris trauma/hemorrhage due to stromal and vascular fragility.

5. Exacerbation or development of uveitic glaucoma via multiple mechanisms (eg, outflow obstruction through trabeculitis/cellular debris/fibrosis, angle closure, neovascularization of the iris, pupillary block).

6. Formation of cyclitic membrane.

7. Hypotony due to postoperative ciliary body shutdown with decreased aqueous production.

8. Postoperative pigment dusting of anterior surface of the IOL: this can lead to loss of best spectacle-corrected visual acuity.

9. IOL explantation for persistent postoperative inflammation (haptic and optic materials).

10. Aphakia.

11. Posterior synechiae: more likely to occur when there is an exuberant postoperative inflammatory response.

12. Anterior capsular contraction with IOL decentration.

13. Posterior capsular fibrosis.

14. Capsular rupture and zonular dehiscence: seen especially in patients with chronic uveitis (ie, Fuchs' heterochromic iridocyclitis).[9]

15. CME: the most common postoperative complication in patients with uveitis.[10,11]

Pertinent History

In addition to the usual ophthalmic history, surgeons should pay particular attention to the following:

1. Appropriate uveitic work-up with established diagnosis and etiology of the uveitis.

2. No history of symptoms suggestive of a uveitic flare-up for at least 2 months.

3. History of glaucoma or uncontrolled IOP.

4. History of rheumatoid arthritis, peripheral ulcerative keratitis, or corneal melts in either eye.

5. Complete list of immunosuppressive medications, including dosage.

Clinical Evaluation

The preoperative evaluation should include a comprehensive eye examination, with consideration of the following points, depending on the specific pathology:

1. Assessment of intraocular inflammation: total control of inflammation = 0 to 2 leukocytes/high-power field (0.2 mm high, narrow slit-beam) in the anterior chamber or vitreous for at least 2 months.[12] Clinically significant inflammation represents 1+ cells (5 to 10 cells/high-power field).[13]

2. Carry out assessment of the cornea via slit lamp, including the presence of band keratopathy, corneal guttata, or keratic precipitates.

3. If the patient has a history of elevated IOP, consider gonioscopy.

4. Perform evaluation of the iris for transillumination defects, neovascularization, anterior or posterior synechiae, or pupillary membranes.

5. Evaluate the lens for phacodonesis or fibrosis of the anterior capsule.

6. Evaluate the adequacy of the red reflex.

7. Careful examination of the vitreous body and posterior segment (macula, retina, and optic nerve) should be performed to assess the integrity of essential structures and the extension of the uveitic process.

IOL Considerations

1. We recommend 100% PMMA PCIOLs in eyes that have a higher risk of anterior capsular contraction. However, foldable IOLs have been used. Definitive long-term data on the safety of these lenses in uveitic patients is not yet available.

2. Heparin surface-modified and acrylic IOLs have been postulated to minimize the corneal edema, anterior chamber reaction, formation of synechia, and IOL deposits. However, over the long-term, the lower incidence of these events has not yet been demonstrated to be statistically significant.

STRATEGIES TO MAXIMIZE OUTCOME

1. To maximize the likelihood of patient satisfaction and promote realistic expectations, discuss any specific risks and complications of cataract surgery that are relevant to the patient.

2. Practice "zero tolerance for inflammation." Total control of inflammation for at least 2 months prior to surgery is essential. Foster et al[14] recommend the following preoperative medications:
   - Three days before surgery use topical 1.0% prednisolone sodium phosphate 4 times a day
   - Two days before surgery use oral prednisone, 1 mg/kg/d (each morning) and oral diflunisal (Dolobid) 500 mg qid or bid.
3. Ensure good control of IOP.
4. Continue preoperative immunosuppressive agents.

PERIOPERATIVE CONSIDERATIONS AND TECHNIQUES

Immediate Preoperative Medications

Maximize preoperative pupillary dilation with the following medications: Phenylephrine 2.5% to 10%, tropicamide 1%, cyclopentolate 0.5 to 1%, and flurbiprofen 0.03% or ketorolac tromethamine 0.5% every 10 minutes x 3, starting 1 hour prior to surgery.

Anesthesia Considerations

General anesthesia should be employed in children and in noncooperative patients, because the surgery can be lengthy and unpredictable. Otherwise, a peribulbar or retrobulbar block can be used. Dependence upon only topical and intracameral anesthesia should be avoided because of the likelihood of extensive iris manipulation.

Wound Construction

A small, clear-corneal incision can be safely performed in patients with uveitis. However, a scleral tunnel approach should be considered if conversion to extracapsular extraction is likely or if the patient has a history of rheumatoid arthritis, peripheral ulcerative keratitis, or corneal melts in either eye.

Pupillary Considerations

A small pupil is a very common finding in the uveitic cataract due to synechial adhesions. In order to maximize pupil dilation and adequate access to the lens, any iris adhesions to the anterior capsule should be carefully broken with a Y-hook, Sinskey hook, or a similar type of instrument inserted through the paracentesis incision at the beginning of the procedure. Once freed from the anterior capsule, the iris can be further dilated using different procedures such as iris hooks, bimanual stretching, radial iridotomy or sphincterectomies (Figure 5-1). Also refer to Chapter 3.

Capsulorrhexis and Other Capsular Considerations

1. An anterior capsulotomy can often be performed using the standard technique. However, one should be alert for increased capsular fragility, fibrotic capsular bands, and calcification of the anterior capsule, all of which can make this technique more difficult. If fibrotic bands or calcific plaques in the anterior capsule present difficulties, capsulotomy scissors (ie, angled Gills scissors) can

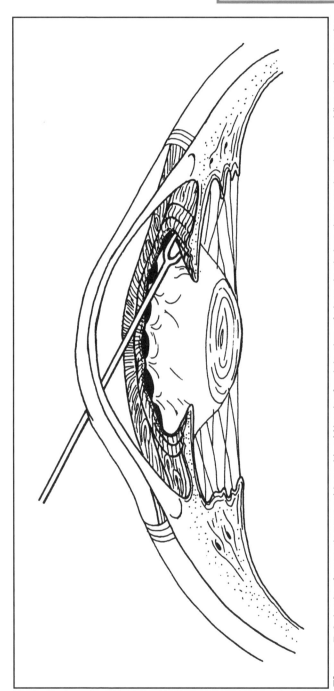

Figure 5-1. Lysis of posterior synechiae with a Y-hook after injection of viscoelastic into the anterior chamber. Viscoelastic can be used to tent the iris and allow better visibility of iris adhesions.

be used to incise them. Be prepared to convert to a can-opener capsulotomy if difficulties arise during the creation of the rhexis. Phacoemulsification often can be completed safely through a can-opener capsulotomy.

2. Since capsular contraction syndrome is more common in uveitic patients,[15] a large, well-centered capsulorrhexis is recommended. Foster proposes a 6-mm capsulorrhexis to minimize this complication. A larger rhexis also facilitates cortical and epithelial clean-up during irrigation and aspiration and therefore prevents lens-induced uveitic aggravation.[16]

Phacoemulsification

Phacoemulsification can be helpful in the uveitic patient due to the advantages of a smaller incision and a shorter surgical time. Heger et al[8] have made the observation that this procedure decreases the inflammatory response, probably due to reduced surgical trauma. Any of the standard phacoemulsification techniques can be used to remove the cataract; however, a chopping technique may be preferred over a nuclear fractis technique depending upon lens density and capsular integrity.

Cortical Aspiration

Thorough removal of cortical material is essential. This is especially important in uveitic patients since any retained cortical material leads to a higher probability of developing severe postoperative inflammation. Similarly, retained lens epithelium can lead to anterior capsular contraction syndrome and posterior capsular opacification.

Special Techniques

Capsular Polishing

- A diamond-dusted capsular polisher can be used to remove residual lens epithelium from the underside of the anterior capsulorrhexis rim and from the posterior capsule. Residual cortical strands can be removed at the same time (Figures 5-2 and 5-3).

Surgical Iridectomy

- A surgical iridectomy should be considered whenever there is a risk of pupillary block, such as in eyes with posterior synechiae. This is done to prevent acute glaucoma (iris bombé) if occlusio pupillae develops.

IOL Implantation

The general consensus among uveitis experts is that in-the-bag PCIOL placement can be performed safely in uveitic patients, provided that the uveitis has been well-controlled for at least 2 months prior to surgery.[2] This has been demonstrated in patients with VKH syndrome, intermediate uveitis, sarcoidosis, and rheumatoid arthritis.[6,7,11,17]

Avoid using IOLs in patients with systemic diseases characterized by chronic inflammation (eg, juvenile rheumatoid arthritis [JRA] associated uveitis).[17,18] The formation of fibrotic membranes in these eyes causes distortion of the pupil and dis-

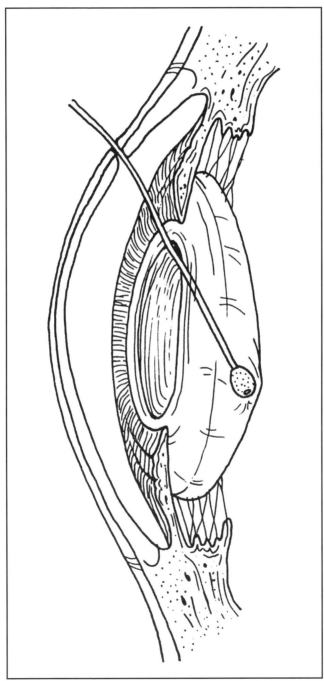

Figure 5-2. Posterior capsular polishing is performed after irrigation/aspiration using a diamond-dusted or sand-blasted irrigating cannula.

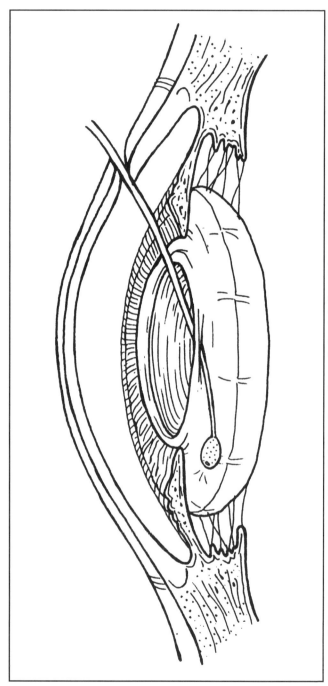

Figure 5-3. Anterior capsular polishing. Polishing is performed after inflation of the capsular bag with viscoelastic to prevent inadvertent posterior capsular damage.

location of the IOL.[2] IOL implantation should also be avoided in patients who have poorly controlled ocular inflammatory conditions, especially those involving the intermediate segment of the eye.[18]

RELEVANT POSTOPERATIVE ISSUES

Complications

1. The most common complications seen in the early postoperative period are:[19]
   - Uveitis 31% (14% severe)
   - Glaucoma 24% (10% requiring extensive antiglaucoma treatment)
   - Pigmented deposits on the anterior surface of the IOL

2. The most common complication in the late postoperative period is posterior capsular opacification.[19]

3. Fifty percent of patients with chronic uveitis develop visually significant CME after cataract surgery.

4. Massive fibrinoid reaction occurs in patients with exuberant postoperative inflammation. Intracameral tPA effectively induces fibrinolysis (a single injection of 10 mcg in 0.1 mm).[20]

5. Postoperative hypotony occurs most commonly in patients with JRA-associated uveitis. Hypotony will usually resolve in several weeks without treatment, unless it is caused by a cyclitic membrane. Hypotony caused by a cyclitic membrane may require secondary surgeries such as pars plana vitrectomy.

Postoperative Medications

1. Aggressive postoperative treatment of inflammation is absolutely necessary. This should include the following:
   - Topical steroid (ie, 1% prednisolone acetate every 1 to 2 hours with slow taper). Additional topical NSAIDs 4x/day should be considered.
   - Transseptal injection of triamcinolone (40 mg of a 40 mg/ml solution). This may be given for immediate results.
   - Oral prednisone. Oral steroids may be needed for those patients who do not have an adequate response to topical steroids and NSAIDs. The starting dose of oral prednisone should be 1 mg/kg/day given as a single dose (observe the standard medical precautions when using high-dose steroids). The tapering schedule depends upon the presence of intraocular inflammation.
   - Diflunisal or other NSAIDs. Use for 2 months unless macular edema develops postoperatively.

2. Continuation of preoperative systemic immunosuppressive medications (observe the standard medical precautions when using immunosuppressive medications). Adjustment of dosage may be needed if inflammation is not under control.

Follow-Up

1. Early evaluation for posterior segment inflammation and CME is recommended so that early treatment can be initiated (see Appendix C).

2. Evaluate the IOL for surface pigment deposits and posterior capsule opacification. Nd:YAG IOL dusting and posterior capsulotomy may be required for decreased visual acuity.

3. Amblyopia therapy may be necessary for proper visual rehabilitation for patients with JRA-associated uveitis who are in the amblyogenic age group.

WHEN TO CONSIDER ALTERNATIVE PROCEDURES

1. For active pars planitis or vitritis: pars plana vitrectomy should be performed at the time of cataract surgery for therapeutic or diagnostic purposes, especially if diagnosis of the uveitis is in question.

2. For uncontrolled glaucoma despite maximal medical treatment, consider performing a combined procedure with shunting device (Ahmed valve) since filtering procedures are less likely to be successful due to inflammation and fibrosis.

3. An ECCE should be performed in eyes with extensive zonular compromise and lens instability to reduce the risk of vitreous loss and dropped nucleus.

KEY POINTS

1. Practice zero tolerance for inflammation.

2. Assess uveitic damage to all ocular structures.

3. Determine etiology of uveitis (if possible).

4. Assess the pupil. Prepare for iris adhesions and a small pupil.

5. Create a large, central capsulorrhexis (6 mm).

6. Perform thorough cortical clean-up and capsular polishing.

7. Avoid IOL placement in the following circumstances:
   - Systemic diseases with chronic inflammation (eg, JRA and others).[18]
   - Chronic ocular inflammatory conditions involving the intermediate segment of the eye.[18]

8. Monitoring closely for postoperative CME.

9. Evaluate postoperative inflammation and adjust immunosuppressive medications in order to maintain zero tolerance to inflammation.

REFERENCES

1. Heiligenhaus A, Foerster M, Wessing A. Long-term results of pars plana vitrectomy in the management of complicated uveitis. *Br J Ophthalmol.* 1994;78:549-554.

2. Rojas B. Cataract surgery in patients with uveitis. *Curr Opin Ophthalmol.* 1996;7(1):11-16.

3. Kijlstra A. The role of cytokines in ocular inflammation. *Br J Ophthalmol.* 1994;78:885-887.

4. Fisher RF. The lens in uveitis. *Trans Ophthalmol Soc UK*. 1981;101:317-320.

5. Marak GE, Scott JM, Duque R, et al. Antioxidant modulation of phacoantigenic endophthalmitis. *Ophthalmic Res*. 1985;17:279-301.

6. Akova YA. Cataract surgery in patients with sarcoidosis-associated uveitis. *Ophthalmology*. 1994;101:473-479.

7. Moorthy RS, Smith RE, Rao NA, et al. Incidence and management of cataracts in Vogh-Koyanagi-Harada syndrome. *Am J Ophthalmol*. 1994;118:197-204.

8. Heger H, Haaskjold E. Cataract surgery with implantation of IOL in patients with uveitis. *Acta Ophthalmol Copenh*. 1994;72:478-482.

9. Barret BT, Eustace P. Clinical comparison of three techniques for evaluating visual function behind cataract. *Eye*. 1995;9:722-727.

10. Tabbara K. Cataract extraction in patients with chronic posterior uveitis. *Int Ophthalmol Clin*. 1995;35:121-131.

11. Forster D, Smith R. Cataract extraction in intermediate uveitis. *Dev Ophthalmol*. 1992;23:204-211.

12. Hooper PL, Rao NA, Smith RE. Cataract extraction in uveitis patients. *Surv Ophthalmol*. 1990;35:120-144.

13. Hogan MJ, Thygeson P. Signs and symptoms of uveitis. *Am J Ophthalmol*. 1959;47:155-170.

14. Foster CS, Meisler DM, Zakov ZN. Extracapsular cataract extraction and posterior chamber lens implantation in uveitis patients. *Ophthalmol*. 1992;99:1234-1241.

15. Davidson JA. Capsule contraction syndrome. *J Cataract Refract Surg*. 1993;19:582-589.

16. Foster CS. Cataract surgery in the patient with uveitis. *Am Acad Ophthalmol Focal Points*. 1994;12:1-6.

17. Matsuo T, Matsou N. Inflammation after cataract extraction and intraocular lens implantation in patients with rheumatoid arthritis. *Am J Ophthalmol*. 1995;114:708-714.

18. Harper SL, Foster CS. Intraocular lens explantation in uveitis. *Int Ophthalmol Clin*. 2000;40(1):107-116.

19. Ram J, Pandav S, Gupta A, et al. Postoperative complications of intraocular lens implantation in patients with Fuchs' heterochromic cylclitis. *J Cataract Refract Surg*. 1995;21:548-551.

20. Heiligenhaus A, Steinmetz B, Lapuente R, et al. Recombinant tissue plasminogen activator in cases with fibrin formation after cataract surgery: a prospecive randomised multicentre study. *Br J Ophthalmol*. 1998;82(7):810-815.

6

PHACOEMULSIFICATION AFTER GLAUCOMA FILTRATION SURGERY

Theresa C. Chen, MD
Victor L. Perez, MD
Susannah G. Rowe, MD, MPH
Roberto Pineda II, MD

RELEVANT PREOPERATIVE ISSUES

Clinical Settings

Visually significant cataracts are common in patients who have undergone glaucoma procedures. Twenty-three to 46% of patients who have had trabeculectomies eventually undergo cataract extraction.[1-3] Of these patients, 94% have cataract surgery within the first 10 years after initial trabeculectomy.[4] Cataract surgery, however, can cause a filter to fail or may result in a 2 to 5 mmHg rise in IOP.[5-6] Nevertheless, there is some evidence to suggest that the rate of bleb failure may be lower for phacoemulsification than for ECCE.[7] Since bleb failure is common after cataract surgery, special consideration must be given to preserving the functioning bleb and maintaining long-term control of IOP after cataract surgery.

Risks and Complications

Patients with previous glaucoma surgery may have greater incidences of the following complications:

1. Complete or partial bleb failure.

2. Bleb trauma during surgery with hypotony and shallowing of the anterior chamber.

3. Early or late postoperative IOP elevations. Postoperative IOP elevation (greater than or equal to 15 mmHg) occurs more commonly in patients with glaucoma (23% to 40%) compared to patients without glaucoma (3%). [8-10]

4. Progression of glaucomatous damage due to poorly controlled postoperative IOP.

5. Endophthalmitis.

Pertinent History

In addition to the usual ophthalmic history, surgeons should pay particular attention to the following:

1. Type and stage of glaucoma.
2. Target IOP.
3. History of previous intraocular surgeries (eg, other failed blebs, etc).
4. The age of the current bleb.
5. History of complications during cataract extraction in the fellow eye.
6. Glaucoma medications, especially miotics (ie, pilocarpine and carbachol).

Clinical Evaluation

The preoperative evaluation should include a comprehensive eye examination, with consideration of the following points, depending on the specific pathology:

1. Bleb size and location. Look for signs of active filtration.
2. IOP measurement.
3. Evaluation of the cornea for signs of endothelial dysfunction (due to previous intraocular surgery).
4. Keratometry to determine degree and axis of astigmatism.
5. Assessment of maximal pupillary dilation; may be limited secondary to synechiae, long-term miotic use, or pseudoexfoliation.
6. Gonioscopy with evaluation of the sclerostomy site.
7. Evaluation of the type of cataract and lens density.
8. Assessment of the optic nerve (fundoscopy and visual field evaluation).

STRATEGIES TO MAXIMIZE OUTCOMES

1. To maximize patient satisfaction and promote realistic expectations, discuss any specific risks and complications of cataract surgery listed under the Risks and Complications section (eg, the possibility of bleb failure) that are relevant to your patient.
2. Wait at least 12 months after performing glaucoma surgery before performing cataract surgery.
3. Control of intraocular inflammation is important to prevent bleb failure. Some authors suggest preoperatively discontinuing miotics or sympathomimetics to minimize postoperative inflammation. Always use topical steroids postoperatively.
4. Develop a plan for pupillary dilation if necessary.
5. Plan a site for clear cornea incision to minimize postoperative astigmatism.
6. If the patient is on phospholine iodide, discontinue use 3 weeks prior to surgery.

PERIOPERATIVE CONSIDERATIONS AND TECHNIQUES

Immediate Preoperative Medications

1. Maximize preoperative pupillary dilation with the following medications: phenylephrine 2.5% to 10%, plus tropicamide 1% or cyclopentolate 0.5% to 1%, and flurbiprofen 0.03% or ketorolac tromethamine 0.5% every 10 minutes x 3, starting 1 hour prior to surgery.[11]

Anesthesia Considerations

1. Avoid unnecessary pressure to the globe after administering anesthesia. Avoid a Honan balloon or Super-Pinky due to potential bleb trauma. Gentle digital massage away from the bleb may be used if the eye pressure seems elevated after peribulbar or retrobulbar block.

2. A peribulbar or retrobulbar block, or topical anesthesia can be used. If using a peribulbar injection, avoid ballooning of the conjunctiva, especially at the bleb site. Intracameral anesthesia should be avoided if extensive iris manipulation is anticipated.

Wound Construction

1. A clear corneal incision is preferred to preserve conjunctiva for future bleb revisions and to lessen intraocular inflammation.

2. Position the cataract wound as far from the functioning bleb as is feasible (Figure 6-1). A temporal or inferotemporal incision is best. Avoid direct bleb or conjunctival trauma. Do not use scleral fixation techniques when making the clear corneal incision. We recommend anchoring the globe by utilizing the paracentesis site to make the clear corneal incision.

3. If a scleral tunnel is necessary, be careful to preserve the conjunctiva as much as possible for future blebs. Handle the conjunctiva as little as possible to lessen surgical trauma. Make a small conjunctival peritomy and achieve meticulous hemostasis. Avoid toothed forceps and employ Hoskins forceps if possible. A scleral tunnel can be placed temporally if necessary.

4. Make sure the wound is relatively snug to help maintain a stable anterior chamber and prevent shallowing and hypotony, which can endanger the bleb.

Viscoelastic Considerations

Choose a high molecular weight cohesive viscoelastic (eg, Healon, Healon GV, or ProVisc) that is easily removed via irrigation and aspiration in order to prevent retained viscoelastic at the sclerostomy site.

Pupillary Considerations

If the pupillary diameter is no greater than 4.0 mm after maximal pharmacological treatment and viscoelastic agents, consider surgically enlarging the pupil prior to the capsulorrhexis (see Chapter 3). However, it is important to avoid excessive iris trauma since the bleb will be endangered by intraocular inflammation, iris debris, and hemorrhage.

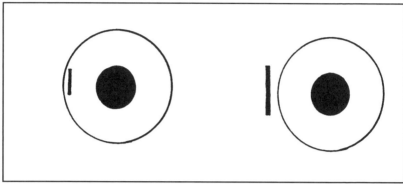

Figure 6-1. A temporal clear corneal incision (left) or scleral tunnel (right) may be the preferred approach in patients with functioning blebs.

Capsulorrhexis and Other Capsular Considerations

An anterior capsulotomy can often be performed using the standard technique. Before initiating the capsulorrhexis, some surgeons instill viscoelastic at the sclerostomy site. This technique may prevent egress of cortical material or lens capsular fragments through the sclerostomy. For the same reason, take care to remove the entire anterior capsular after capsulorrhexis.

Hydrodissection

Hydrodissection and hydrodelineation can be performed using the standard technique.

Phacoemulsification

Any of the standard phacoemulsification techniques can be used to remove the cataract. However, if the pupil remains small after pupil dilation, a nuclear chopping technique may be preferred over a nuclear fractis technique depending upon lens density and capsular integrity.

Cortical Aspiration

Thorough cortical cleanup should be performed after phacoemulsification to minimize postoperative inflammation, which can endanger the bleb. If the pupil is small, a Kuglen hook or Y-hook can be used to retract the pupil and allow direct visualization of any remaining cortical material. Be careful to prevent migration of cortical material into the sclerostomy site. It is important to maintain constant pressure in the anterior chamber throughout the entire procedure to prevent damage to the bleb. Do not permit collapse of the bleb due to prolonged hypotony since it may not reopen after the surgery.

IOL Implantation

1. A foldable posterior chamber IOL should be implanted if at all possible, preferably through a small clear corneal incision.

2. Although an anterior chamber IOL should be avoided if the angle is compromised, it is not necessarily contraindicated in the presence of glaucoma. The newer semiflexible, open-loop anterior chamber IOL may be a safe alternative in patients whose intraoperative conditions are not conducive to a sutured lens or for those in which the surgeon is uncomfortable with the procedure. The lens haptics should not be near the sclerostomy.

3. Meticulous aspiration of viscoelastic is necessary to prevent occlusion of the bleb and to avoid postoperative IOP spikes.

4. Assessment of bleb function and integrity is performed by instilling a balanced salt solution into the anterior chamber and watching for ballooning of the bleb.

5. Consider placing a 10-0 nylon suture at the wound if digital massage is anticipated for bleb maintenance.

Special Techniques: Bleb Revision

If the bleb does not appear to be functioning at the conclusion of the cataract surgery, bleb revision may be needed. A cyclodialysis spatula may be gently passed through the anterior chamber into the sclerostomy site, and adhesions can be carefully lysed. If the sclerostomy contains retained nuclear or cortical material, a Simcoe cannula can be used to aspirate the debris. The irrigation tube can be manually occluded if necessary to prevent washing the material further into the sclerostomy.

Immediate Postoperative Medications

Subconjunctival steroid injections may be given, placed as far away from the bleb as possible. If a miotic is given, intracameral Miostat (Alcon, Fort Worth, Tex) (carbachol) may also reduce the incidence and severity of postoperative IOP rises. Miochol (Alcon, Fort Worth, Tex) (acetylcholine) does not provide long-acting IOP control.

RELEVANT POSTOPERATIVE ISSUES

Complications

1. IOP spikes due to retained viscoelastic or compromised bleb functioning.
2. Steroid-induced IOP elevations (more common in patients with glaucoma).
3. Bleb failure.
4. Postoperative inflammation, especially when extensive iris manipulation has been performed.
5. Blebitis, endophthalmitis.

Postoperative Medications

1. Frequent steroid drops may be needed every 1 to 2 hours while awake, especially if there is significant postoperative inflammation, bleeding, or residual cortical or particulate material. They may also be used longer than usual to prevent bleb failure.

2. Early cycloplegia. This may not be as critical in pseudophakic patients, as anterior chamber shallowing and choroidals are not as common as in phakic or aphakic patients.

3. Topical antibiotics.

4. May need adjunctive 5-Fluorouracil (5-FU) in 5 mg doses (0.1 ml of 5FU 50 mg/ml) subconjunctivally 180 degrees away from the bleb; may be used once or twice a week or more often.

Follow-Up

1. Close follow-up is important for monitoring the IOP.

2. Monitor the integrity of the bleb. If the function of the bleb is in question, consider gentle digital massage.

WHEN TO CONSIDER ALTERNATIVE PROCEDURES

1. Poor IOP control or a patient on two or more glaucoma medications. Consider a concomitant glaucoma procedure.

2. Failing or failed bleb. Consider bleb revision or another glaucoma procedure prior to cataract surgery.

3. Pseudoexfoliation with significant zonular instability. Consider postponing surgery. These patients have more postoperative inflammation and should understand the increased risks of bleb failure as well as risks with cataract surgery.

KEY POINTS

1. Delay cataract surgery until the bleb has matured (at least 1 year).

2. Assess bleb function before surgery.

3. Evaluate pupillary dilation.

4. Minimize conjunctival trauma.

5. Utilize a small clear corneal incision far from the bleb (temporal if possible).

6. Assess bleb function upon completion of cataract extraction and revise if needed.

7. Aggressively treat postoperative inflammation and IOP spikes.

REFERENCES

1. Nouri-Mahdavi K, Brigatti L, Weitzman M, et al. Outcomes of trabeculectomy for primary open-angle glaucoma. Ophthalmology. 1995;102:1760-1769.

2. Araujo SV, Spaeth GL, Roth SM, et al. A ten-year follow-up on a prospective, randomized trial of postoperative corticosteroids after trabeculectomy. Ophthalmology. 1995;102:1753-1759.

3. Popovic V, Sjostrand J. Long-term outcome following trabeculectomy: I. Retrospective analysis of IOP regulation and cataract formation. Acta Ophthalmol Copenh. 1991;69:299-304.

4. Chen TC, Wilensky JT, Viana MAG. Long-term follow-up of initial trabeculectomy. *Ophthalmology.* 1997;104:1120-1125.

5. Schuman JS. Surgical management of coexisting cataract and glaucoma. *Ophthalmic Surg Lasers.* 1996,; 27: 45-59.

6. Savage JA, Thomas JV, Belcher CD, et al. Extracapsular cataract extraction and posterior chamber intraocular lens implantation in glaucomatous eyes. *Ophthalmology.* 1985; 92: 1506-1516.

7. Seah SK, Jap A, Prata JA Jr, et al. Cataract surgery after trabeculectomy. *Ophthalmic Surg Lasers.* 1996;27(7):587-594.

8. Tomey KF, Traverso CE. The glaucomas in aphakia and pseudophakia. *Surv Ophthalmol.* 1991;36:79-112.

9. McCartney DL, Memmen JE, Stark WJ, et al. The efficacy and safety of combined trabeculectomy, cataract extraction, and intraocular lens implantation. *Ophthalmology.* 1988;95:754-763.

10. Ruderman JM, Fundingsland B, Meyer MA. Combined phacoemulsification and trabeculectomy with mitomycin C. *J Cataract Refract Surg.* 1996;22:1085-1090.

11. Solomon KD, Turkalj JW, Whiteside SB, et al. Topical 0.5% Ketorolac vs. 0.03% Flubiprofen for inhibition of miosis during cataract surgery. *Arch Ophthalmol.* 1997;115:1119-1122.

7

THE SHORT EYE

Sandra L. Cramer, MD
Victor L. Perez, MD
Susannah G. Rowe, MD, MPH
Roberto Pineda II, MD

RELEVANT PREOPERATIVE ISSUES

Clinical Settings

A short or small eye is defined as an eye with an axial length of less than 22.5 mm. Eyes of this length are almost always hyperopic. The short eye may be associated with a shallow anterior chamber, which is defined as a depth of less than 2 mm. These eyes have a higher risk of narrow-angle glaucoma with acute, intermittent, and chronic angle closure and may have refractive amblyopia.

There are many differing nomenclatures that have been used to categorize short eyes. Listed below is one recently published classification system:[1]

1. Simple micropthalmos (nanophthalmos): this is a small version of a normal eye with normal proportions.

   - Average refraction: +13.60 D
   - Total axial length: <20.5 mm
   - Average total axial length: 17.0 mm
   - Associated with pseudoexfoliation (PXF) and glaucoma[2]
   - More common in females

2. Complex microphthalmos: this condition is defined as microphthalmos with other associated intraocular anomalies, systemic diseases, or syndromes.

3. Relative anterior microphthalmos (RAM) or anterior microphthalmos: RAM is a simple, isolated, idiopathic microphthalmos. In this condition, the axial length is normal but the anterior segment is disproportionately small. Approximately 20% of eyes with an axial length of less than 21 mm have RAM. These eyes have the following characteristics:

- Horizontal corneal diameter: <11 mm
- Total axial length (TAL): >20 mm
- Average TAL: 21.98 mm
- AC depth: 2 mm (approximately)
- Average refraction: -0.13 D
- Associated with PXF and glaucoma

4. Microcornea:
- Corneal horizontal diameter: <11 mm
- Multiple malformations are frequent

Risks and Complications

Patients with short eyes may have greater incidences of the following complications:

1. Iris trauma/prolapse.

2. Corneal edema.

3. Pupillary block (iris bombé).

4. Choroidal effusion (uveal effusion syndrome).

5. Aqueous misdirection (malignant glaucoma).

6. Expulsive hemorrhage.

7. Postoperative inflammation.

Pertinent History

In addition to the usual ophthalmic history, surgeons should pay particular attention to the following:

1. Glaucoma: history of narrow angle, prior laser iridotomy, miotic use.

2. Previous ocular surgery, especially glaucoma filtration surgery.

3. Hyperopia.

4. Amblyopia.

5. Complications during cataract surgery in the fellow eye.

Clinical Evaluation

The preoperative evaluation should include a comprehensive eye examination, with consideration of the following points, depending on the specific pathology:

1. Compare the refractive error of the fellow eye and determine the need for future cataract surgery in that eye. This will help to determine the final target refraction for the eye undergoing surgery.

2. Evaluate for prominent brows and deepset eyes.

3. Examine endothelium for the presence of guttata or other endothelial pathology.

4. Determine anterior chamber depth.

5. Perform gonioscopy to evaluate for narrow angles or iris bombé.

6. Determine degree of pupillary dilation.

7. Evaluate for signs of pseudoexfoliation.

8. Observe for anterior or posterior synechiae secondary to narrow-angle glaucoma.

9. Repeat biometry (A-scan) until consistent, reproducible axial length measurements are obtained. Measure the fellow eye to compare axial lengths. Consider submersion biometry and B-scan in these cases, as well as the new biometric laser interferometry (IOL Master by Zeiss/Humphrey, Jena, Germany).

10. Use of the Hoffer-Q[3] or Holladay II[4] formula is recommended for axial lengths <22 mm. Do not use empirical, regression-based formulas for short eyes due to inaccuracies (second-generation IOL formulas).

STRATEGIES TO MAXIMIZE OUTCOMES

1. To maximize patient satisfaction and promote realistic expectations, discuss any specific risks and complications of cataract surgery listed in the Risks and Complications section that are relevant to your patient.

2. If considering piggyback IOLs, discuss appropriate risks and postoperative refractive outcomes.

3. Review with the patient the possible need for glasses or second surgery (ie, piggyback IOL placement), postoperative IOL exchange, or laser refractive surgery to correct residual refractive error.

4. Discontinue any miotic agent at least 3 days prior to surgery. Pay special attention to phosphylene iodide, which should be discontinued 2 to 3 weeks before surgery.

5. After consultation with the patient's internist, stop aspirin, oral NSAIDs, and other anticoagulants such as gingko biloba 10 days prior to surgery due to risk of iris bleeding, particularly if extensive iris manipulation is anticipated.

6. Consider cyclopentolate 1% or scopolamine 0.25% one to two drops bid 3 days prior to surgery if there is evidence of a small pupil or history of uveitis.

7. Consider preoperative topical steroids and nonsteroidal agents to minimize postoperative inflammation if there is a history of uveitis (one to two drops qid 3 days preoperatively).

8. Consider performing a preoperative laser peripheral iridotomy if the AC angle is occludable.

IOL Considerations

1. Use an IOL with a 6.0-mm optic or larger if the pupil will need to be surgically enlarged.

2. Consider Heparin surface-modified IOLs if extensive iris manipulation is needed.

Special Note: Piggyback Lenses

1. Controversy has surrounded the use of piggyback lenses since they were first described in 1993 by Dr. Gayton.[5] Holladay, Gills, and others report successfully using piggyback lenses for high hyperopes.[6,7] Prior to using two or three IOLs simultaneously, review the literature and formulate your surgical strategy.

2. Consider using the Holladay II formula for piggyback IOLs (Holladay IOL Consultant Software, Holladay Consulting, Inc., Bellaire, TX).[6] Some surgeons divide the total required power equally between the two implants. Others advocate placing two-thirds of the total power in the posterior implant since it may be more stable and, therefore, less likely to cause optical aberrations due to shifting.

3. Interlenticular opacification (ILO) or interpseudophakos opacification (IPO) is a late complication of piggyback IOLs that has recently been described.[8,9] ILO consists of lens epithelial cell ingrowth within the interface between the two IOLs. Laminin (a basement membrane component) has been implicated in the formation of ILO. This condition can result in decreased best-corrected visual acuity, as well as hyperopic shifts. ILO occurs more commonly when using two acrylic IOLs (Figure 7-1).

4. PMMA optics are not as thick as acrylic optics; therefore, two IOLs fit more easily together in the capsular bag.

PERIOPERATIVE CONSIDERATIONS AND TECHNIQUES

Immediate Preoperative Medications

To maximize pupillary dilation, use phenylephrine 2.5% to 10% plus tropicamide 1% or cyclopentolate 0.5% to 1%, and flurbiprofen 0.03% or ketorolac promethamine 0.5% every 10 minutes x 3, 1 hour before surgery.

Anesthesia Considerations

We recommend local anesthesia in these cases. Topical/intracameral anesthesia is not our first choice due to the greater risk of iris prolapse and trauma. Additionally, local anesthesia facilitates dealing with intraoperative complications. Because local anesthesia can increase retrobulbar pressure, ocular compression (with digital massage or a device such as a Honan balloon or Super-Pinky) is advocated.

Wound Construction

Patients with deepset eyes and prominent brows may require a temporal approach. In general, we advocate the use of long scleral tunnels. Clear corneal incisions may be performed but will be problematic because of the higher incidence of corneal edema and iris prolapse. Additionally, a clear corneal incision may take up a larger percentage of the small cornea in these cases. Therefore, avoid a clear corneal incision if the corneal diameter is <10 mm or the axial length is <18 mm. Instead, make a relatively long scleral tunnel to prevent iris prolapse through the wound. Make sure the tunnel is relatively snug to help maintain a stable anterior chamber and prevent further shallowing.

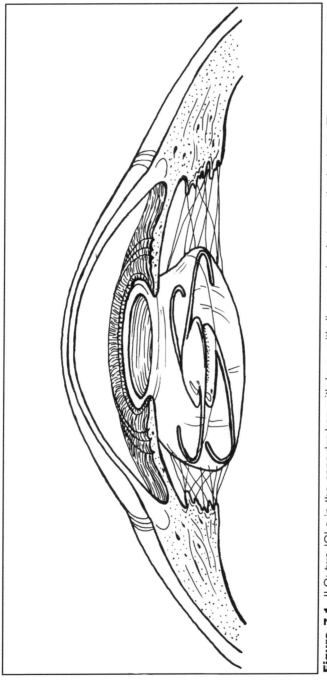

Figure 7-1. ILO: two IOLs in the capsular bag with lens epithelium growing between the implants. There is posterior displacement of the lenses with hyperopic shift.

Finally, a clear corneal technique may not be possible if the eye is very hyperopic, since highly hyperopic patients often require very high-powered IOL implants. These IOLs are currently only available with rigid optics and require a larger incision.

Viscoelastic Considerations

Use generous amounts of a viscodispersive viscoelastic with high coatability (<1 million Daltons [Viscoat]) to protect the corneal endothelium from mechanical trauma and to absorb phacoemulsification energy. Consider using the "soft shell viscoelastic technique" as described by Dr. S. Arshinoff.[10] Inject a small amount of viscodispersive viscoelastic first to coat the endothelium. Then, inject a second high molecular weight, highly cohesive viscoelastic (ProVisc, Healon, Healon GV, or Amvisc Plus) just above the lens capsule to push the first viscoelastic against the endothelium and to maintain the anterior chamber. Additional cohesive viscoelastic placed over the anterior capsule and proximal iris may be helpful before the capsulorrhexis to minimize the potential for iris prolapse (see Appendix E).

Pupillary Considerations

A well-dilated pupil is essential since the diameter of the hyperopic anterior segment may be small and may not allow a reasonably sized capsulorrhexis. Additional pupillary dilation may be required (see Chapter 3).

Capsulorrhexis and Other Capsular Considerations

If a piggyback IOL is planned, consider creating a 7-mm capsulorrhexis to lessen the risk of ILO.

Phacoemulsification

With hyperopic/nanophthalmic eyes, it is crucial to maintain adequate pressurization of the eye throughout the procedure to minimize choroidal effusions. Elevate the bottle height to help maintain anterior pressure. It is best to phacoemulsify the nucleus in the endocapsular bag to minimize endothelial trauma. If a small pupil requires the use of iris hooks, place iris retractors during the capsulorrhexis only; remove them before phacoemulsification to provide as deep an anterior chamber as possible. Iris hooks may shallow the anterior chamber during phacoemulsification.

Cortical Aspiration

Meticulous cleanup of cortical material and anterior capsular polishing may reduce the likelihood of interlenticular opacification in the case of piggyback IOLs.

IOL Implantation (Piggyback IOLs)

Surgeons suggest two strategies to minimize the risk of ILO: one can either place the first lens in the bag and the second in the sulcus, or create a very large (7 mm) capsulorrhexis, which lessens contact between the IOLs and the anterior capsule. Meticulous cortical aspiration, especially at the lens equator, and anterior capsular polishing may reduce the incidence of interlenticular opacification.[11] It has been recommended that haptic-configured IOLs are aligned in the same orientation, while plate-configured IOLs are oriented 90 degrees from each other.

Special Techniques for Intraoperative Complications

1. For intraoperative pupillary block, consider a surgical peripheral iridectomy or postponing the surgery until the next day.

2. Choroidal effusions. Options include discontinuing the surgery and reoperating when the IOP is controlled, draining the choroidals, or pars plana vitrectomy.

3. Ciliolenticular block (also called ciliary block, malignant glaucoma, or aqueous misdirection). Consider discontinuing the surgery until the IOP is controlled or performing a pars plana vitrectomy.

Immediate Posoperative Medications

Use a subconjunctival injection of dexamethisone 20 to 40 mg immediately following cataract surgery to minimize postoperative inflammation due to excess phaco power nearer to the corneal endothelium.

RELEVANT POSTOPERATIVE ISSUES

Complications

1. Refractive error and anisometropia. Once the refraction of the operated eye is stable, perform surgery on the fellow eye as soon as possible to minimize the period of anisometropia. Early cataract surgery is indicated in the fellow eye for patients with significant anisometropia, since patients will be unlikely to tolerate spectacles due to induced anisokonia and diplopia. Use an IOL implant that provides balanced binocular vision (final refraction of the two eyes should be within 3 D of each other). Once the refraction of the first eye is stable, compare the postoperative refractive result of the first eye to the target refraction. Adjust the IOL choice for the second eye accordingly.

2. Corneal edema. Usually temporary and resolves with standard treatment.

3. Intraocular inflammation. Usually due to iris trauma, may be short-term or chronic. Adjust the postoperative steroid course accordingly.

4. Postoperative glaucoma. May be due to blood debris, pigment, or inflammatory cells in the trabecular meshwork. May require short- or long-term glaucoma medications.

5. Ciliolenticular block (also called ciliary block, malignant glaucoma, or aqueous misdirection). Seen more often in patients with relative anterior microphthalmos (RAM). Predisposing factors include narrow angles and a shallow anterior chamber.

Postoperative Medications

1. Consider intensive treatment with a topical steroid (prednisolone acetate 1% one to two gtts every 1 to 2 hours) due to iris manipulation.

2. Consider NSAIDs (eg, ketorolac 0.5% [Acular] or diclofenac 0.1% [Voltaren]).

Follow-Up

1. Consider more frequent postoperative visits if there is significant corneal edema, uveitis, or IOP rise.

2. Monitor the patient for ciliary and pupillary blocks.

3. An early refraction should be performed to determine if an IOL exchange is needed.

4. If using piggyback IOLs, monitor for IOL decentration.

5. Consider a B-scan if there is a high suspicion of choroidal hemorrhages.

WHEN TO CONSIDER ALTERNATIVE PROCEDURES

1. RAM/complex microphthalmos. Glaucoma may be secondary to underlying associated pathology. It may be difficult to control postoperative pressures, and further glaucoma surgery may be required. Consider a combined cataract surgery and glaucoma procedure.

2. Compromised corneal endothelium. Consider a combined cataract extraction and penetrating keratoplasty.

3. In patients with a history of ciliary block in the other eye, consider combined cataract extraction and pars plana vitrectomy.

4. In eyes with pseudoexfoliation, an anterior chamber depth of less than 2.5 mm is associated with an increased risk for intraoperative complications. Consider ECCE.

KEY POINTS

1. Discuss possible binocular refractive outcomes with patients.

2. Pay careful attention to biometry measurements in comparison to the fellow eye.

3. Use the Holladay II[4] or Hoffer Q[3] formula for IOL power calculations (see Appendix A).

4. Consider using piggyback IOLs for high hyperopia.

5. Consider a prophylactic peripheral iridotomy.

6. Use a scleral tunnel rather than clear corneal incision. Determine the wound size based on the available lens options.

7. Use a temporal approach in patients with prominent brows and deepset eyes.

8. Watch for AC shallowing and ocular pressure increase during surgery. Be prepared for suprachoroidal hemorrhages, choroidal effusions, or pupillary block.

9. Perform an early postoperative refraction.

REFERENCES

1. Auffarth G, Blum M, Faller U, et al. Relative anterior microphthalmos. *Ophthalmology*. 2000;107:1555-1560.

2. Junemann A, Kuchle M, Handel A, et al. Cataract surgery in nanophthalmic eyes with an axial length of less than 20.5 mm. *Klin Monatsbl Augenheilkd*. 1998:212(1)13-22.

3. Hoffer KJ. The Hoffer Q formula: a comparison of theoretic and regression formulas. *J Cataract Refract Surg*. 1993;19(6):700-712.

4. Hoffer KJ. Clinical results using the Holladay II intraocular lens power formula. *J Cataract Refract Surg*. 2000;26(8):1233-1237.

5. Gayton Jl, Sanders VN. Implanting two posterior chamber intraocular lenses in a case of microphthalmos. *J Cataract Refract Surg*. 1993;19(6):776-777.

6. Fenzl RE, Gills JP, Gills JP. Piggyback intraocular lens implantation. *Curr Opin Ophthalmol*. 2000;11:73-76.

7. Holladay JT, Gills JP, Leidlin J, et al. Achieving emmetropia in extremely short eyes with two piggyback lenses. *Ophthalmology*. 1996;103(7):1118-1123.

8. Shugar JK, Keeler S. Interpseudophakos intraocular lens surface opacification as a late complication of piggyback acrylic posterior chamber lens implantation. *J Cataract Refract Surg*. 2000;26(3):448-455.

9. Gayton JL, Apple DJ, Peng Q, et al. Interlenticular opacification: clinicopathological correlation of a complication of posterior chamber piggyback intraocular lenses. *J Cataract Refract Surg*. 2000;26(3):330-336.

10. Arshinoff SA. Dispersive-cohesive visoelastic soft shell technique. *J Cataract Refract Surg*. 1999;25(2):167-173.

11. Chaudry NA, Flynn Jr HW, Murray TG, et al. Pars plana vitrectomy during cataract surgery for prevention of aqueous misdirection in high-risk fellow eyes. *Am J Ophthamol*. 2000;129(3):387-388.

8

THE LONG EYE

Christopher Starr, MD
Victor L. Perez, MD
Roberto Pineda II, MD

RELEVANT PREOPERATIVE ISSUES

Clinical Settings

The long or myopic eye can be defined by a refractive error of at least -6 D, or more accurately by an axial length of more than 26 mm. Nuclear sclerotic cataracts are commonly seen in myopic eyes, and these cataracts tend to develop at a younger age in long eyes. Associated anatomic ocular manifestations include poor pupillary dilatation; deep anterior chamber; wide, deep, flimsy capsular bag; staphyloma; and retinal degeneration. It is reported that approximately 12% of patients with high myopia experience retinal tears and holes.[1,2]

Risks and Complications

Patients with long eyes may have greater incidences of the following complications:

1. Globe perforation with retrobulbar anesthesia.
2. Risk of suprachoroidal hemorrhage (more common in myopic eyes).
3. Decreased accuracy in IOL implant power calculation.
4. Increased risk for posterior capsular rupture and zonular dehiscence.
5. Posterior capsular opacification (50%).[1]
6. Nd:YAG capsulotomy for the treatment of posterior capsular opacification has an increased risk (up to 4x) of retinal detachment.
7. Risk of retinal detachment (RD). Phacoemulsification has the lowest risk of retinal detachment (1%), compared to ECCE (2%) or ICCE (5% to 6%).[1,3]

Pertinent History

In addition to the usual ophthalmic history, surgeons should pay particular attention to the following:

1. History of lattice degeneration, retinal holes, tears, and detachments.

2. Previous retinal surgery.

3. Complications during cataract surgery on the fellow eye.

4. Flashes and floaters.

Clinical Evaluation

The preoperative evaluation should include a comprehensive eye examination, with consideration of the following points, depending on the specific pathology:

1. Compare the refractive error of the fellow eye and determine the need for future cataract surgery in that eye. This will help to determine the final target refraction for the eye undergoing surgery.

2. Consider pupil size, shape, and dilation.

3. Determine the depth of the anterior chamber.

4. Grade the degree and type of lens opacity. In general, mild nuclear sclerotic cataracts will be more visually debilitating in high myopes than in others.

5. Perform a thorough dilated fundus exam with scleral depression to evaluate the presence of subclinical retinal breaks.

6. Repeat biometry (A-scan) until consistent, reproducible axial length measurements are obtained due to the incidence of staphyloma in longer axial length eyes. Measure the fellow eye to compare axial lengths. Consider submersion biometry and B-scan in these cases, as well as the new biometric laser interferometry (IOL Master).

7. The Sanders-Retzlaff-Kraff theoretical (SRK/T) formula has been shown to be more accurate for lens calculations in long eyes.[4]

STRATEGIES TO MAXIMIZE OUTCOMES

1. To maximize patient satisfaction and promote realistic expectations, discuss any specific risks and complications of cataract surgery listed under Risks and Complications that are relevant to your patient. Discuss the risk of retinal detachment and posterior capsular opacification, as well as the possible need for secondary procedures.

2. If the patient is using miotic agents, discontinue use 3 days prior to surgery. If miosis is a potential problem, consider instilling cyclopentolate 1% or scopolamine 0.25% one to two drops bid 3 days before surgery.

3. Due to the high risk of suprachoroidal hemorrhage, all blood thinners should be discontinued prior to surgery, including herbal medications such as ginkgo biloba. If the patient is on anticoagulants, discuss the surgical plan and timing of discontinuing anticoagulants with the patient's internist.

4. Prophylactic laser or cryoretinopexy should be applied, when necessary, prior to phacoemulsification. One study noted that 11% of highly myopic eyes required prophylactic laser treatment for retinal tears prior to the cataract operation.[5]

IOL Considerations

1. IOL choice:

   Choose an optic of at least 6.0 mm. Since long eyes have a large, wide capsular bag, a larger lens is often needed.

   Consider an acrylic lens. These lenses have a lower incidence of posterior capsular opacification. Moreover, since there is a higher chance of future retinal reattachment surgery in myopes (potentially with silicone oil tamponade), a silicone IOL is discouraged.

2. Patients with poor visual potential (such as those with age-related macular degeneration [AMD]) should be left more myopic to improve their near magnification.

PERIOPERATIVE CONSIDERATIONS AND TECHNIQUES

Immediate Preoperative Medications

To maximize pupillary dilation, use phenylephrine 2.5% to 10% plus tropicamide 1% or cyclopentolate 0.5% to 1%, plus flurbiprofen 0.03% or ketorolac promethamine 0.5% every 10 minutes x 3, 1 hour before surgery.

Anesthesia Considerations

If possible, avoid retrobulbar injections because of the increased risk of globe perforation, as long eyes often have thinned scleras. Peri- and parabulbar injections are preferred over retrobulbar injections; however, globe perforation is still possible with these techniques. Be especially careful with patients who have scleral buckles, since they are at a greater risk of inadvertent perforation of the globe due to needle misdirection. For cooperative patients, topical or intracameral anesthesia avoids the risk of globe perforation.

Wound Construction

1. A small clear corneal incision is preferred if possible. However, this technique may not be possible if the eye is very myopic, since highly myopic patients often require very low-power or minus-power IOL implants. These IOLs are currently only available with rigid optics and require a 6-mm incision. Therefore, in these cases a scleral tunnel approach should be used.

2. If a scleral tunnel is used, the incision should be close to the limbus, and the tunnel should not be too long. Such a tunnel will minimize corneal distortion typically caused in myopic eyes when the phacoemulsification instruments are angled more vertically into the deep anterior chamber.

Viscoelastic Considerations

A high viscosity, highly cohesive viscoelastic (eg, Healon, Healon GV, or Amvisc Plus) is useful for inflation and support of the large, floppy capsular bag. It is also useful in maintaining pupillary dilation and hemostasis.

Pupillary Considerations

Since some high myopes dilate poorly, maintain a low threshold for employing pupillary dilation (see Chapter 3).

Capsulorrhexis and Other Capsular Considerations

The ideal capsulorrhexis size is 5 to 6 mm. Since the pupil and crystalline lens are often very large, there can be a tendency to make the capsulorrhexis too large, resulting in radial tears. Measure with calipers if necessary to avoid oversizing the capsulorrhexis. Usually the red reflex is bright in these patients.

Hydrodissection

Thorough hydrodissection is essential to ensure easy nuclear manipulation and complete cortical removal, since patients are often younger and more likely to have capsular adhesions. Use a 26-gauge blunt cannula to elevate the anterior capsular flap away from the cortical material. The cannula will maintain the anterior capsule in a tented-up position at the injection site. To ensure an effective fluid wave, it is important to insert the cannula far enough toward the equator to prevent reflux of fluid along the cannula barrel. Once the cannula is properly placed and the anterior capsule is elevated, continuous irrigation will create a fluid wave and cleave the cortex from the capsule in most locations. Repetition in several quadrants will facilitate complete cortical cleavage.

Phacoemulsification

1. Because of the deep anterior chamber and capsular bag, the phacoemulsification handpiece tip should be angled more than normal (ie, 45 degrees or flared) in order to minimize excessive movement in the eye and distortion of the wound.

2. It is important to maintain constant pressure in the anterior chamber throughout the entire procedure. Because of the responsiveness of the lens-iris diaphragm, rapid fluctuations in pressure can lead to "trampolining" of the posterior capsule with resultant capsular and zonular compromise.

3. Since nuclear sclerotic cataracts are more common in high myopic patients, phacoemulsification energy will often need to be higher than expected when performing initial nuclear sculpting. If the phaco power is not adequate, the extra back-and-forth rocking of the nucleus can lead to capsular compromise or zonular dehiscence. One technique to minimize phacoemulsification energy and nuclear rocking is the phaco-chop technique. Due to the deep anterior chamber, nuclear fragments can safely be emulsified above the iris plane, minimizing trauma to the capsular bag.

IOL Implantation

Large IOLs (6 mm or larger), whether posterior, sulcus, or anterior, are often necessary to ensure a proper fit in the myopic eye. Because of the larger capsular bag, an overall haptic diameter of 13 mm or greater is desired.

RELEVANT POSTOPERATIVE ISSUES

Complications

1. Refractive error and anisometropia. Once the refraction of the operated eye is stable, perform surgery on the fellow eye as soon as possible to minimize the period of anisometropia. Early cataract surgery is indicated in the fellow eye for patients with significant anisometropia, since patients will be unlikely to tolerate spectacles due to induced anisokonia and diplopia. Use an IOL implant that provides balanced binocular vision (final refraction of the two eyes should be within 3 D of each other). Once the refraction of the first eye is stable, compare the postoperative refractive result of the first eye to the target refraction. Adjust the IOL choice for the second eye accordingly.

2. Unanticipated postoperative refractive error. This is more common in high myopes. Early IOL exchange is indicated in these cases.

3. Posterior capsular opacification. This occurs more commonly in myopic eyes. Nd:YAG capsulotomy should be deferred until clinically necessary because of the increased risk of retinal detachment following the procedure (90 days minimum).[6]

4. Retinal tears and detachments. If the surgery was complicated, a dilated retinal examination should be performed within the first week after surgery, ideally within the first 48 hours, especially if the patient complains of photopsias and floaters. If the view of the fundus is obscured by inflammation and/or corneal edema and there is a high clinical suspicion of retinal complications, perform a B-scan.

Postoperative Medications

Consider routine treatment with a topical NSAID (eg, ketorolac 0.5% [Acular] or diclofenac 0.1% [Voltaren]) and topical antibiotics.

Follow-Up

1. An early dilated examination is indicated to evaluate for the presence of retinal tears or detachment.

2. An early refraction should be performed to determine if IOL exchange is needed.

WHEN TO CONSIDER ALTERNATIVE PROCEDURES

1. In patients with previous vitrectomy, consider ECCE in order to decrease risks of zonular and capsular complications due to increased lens-iris diaphragm instability.

KEY POINTS

1. Discuss possible binocular refractive outcomes with patients.

2. Pay careful attention to biometry measurements in comparison to the fellow eye.

3. Use the SRK/T formula for IOL power calculations.

4. Determine wound construction based on the available lens options.

5. Stabilize the AC during phacoemulsification.

6. Perform an early postoperative retinal examination.

REFERENCES

1. Lyle WA, Jin GJ. Phacoemulsification with IOL implantation in high myopia. *J Cataract Refract Surg.* 1996;22(2):238-242.

2. Percival SP. Redefinition of high myopia: the relationship of axial length measurement to pathology and its relevance to cataract surgery. *Dev Ophthalmol.* 1987;14:42-46.

3. Tielsch JM, Leggro MW, Cassard SD, et al. Risk factors for retinal detachment after cataract surgery. A population-based case-control study. *Ophthalmology.* 1996;103(10):1537.

4. Hoffer KJ. Clinical results using the Holladay II intraocular lens power formula. *J Cataract Refract Surg.* 2000;26(8):1233-1237.

5. Fan DSP, Lam DSC, Li KKW. Retinal complications after cataract extraction in patients with high myopia. *Ophthalmology.* 1999;106:688-692.

6. Javitt JC, Vitale S, Canner JK, et al. National outcomes of cataract extraction. Increased risk of retinal complications associated with Nd:YAG laser capsulotomy. The Cataract Patient Outcomes Research Team. *Ophthalmology.* 1992.

SUGGESTED READING

Buratto L. *Phacoemulsification: Principles and Techniques.* Thorofare, NJ: SLACK Incorporated; 1998.

Jaffe NS, Jaffe MS, Jaffe GF. *Cataract Surgery and its Complications.* 6th ed. St. Louis, Mo: CV Mosby; 1997.

9

The Dense Cataract

Sandra L. Cramer, MD
Victor L. Perez, MD
Susannah G. Rowe, MD, MPH

RELEVANT PREOPERATIVE ISSUES

Clinical Settings

A challenge that all phacoemulsification surgeons will face is the dense or brunescent cataract. These cataracts have been associated with advanced age, tobacco use, poor nutrition, and silicone oil. They are usually bilateral, although they can be asymmetric, and often cause a myopic shift. These cases can be complicated due to a limited red reflex, the dense consistency of the nucleus, and the virtual absence of a protective cortical shell. Brunescent and black cataracts may be associated with leathery, cohesive, tenacious fibers: these make division of the nucleus difficult. Dense cataracts are associated with relative shallowing of the AC and narrow angles.

Risks and Complications

Patients with dense cataracts may have greater incidences of the following complications:

1. Inability to complete an anterior capsulorrhexis.
2. Necessity of converting to an ECCE.[1]
3. Corneal or scleral incisional burn.[1]
4. Endothelial damage and corneal edema due to a reduced safety zone between the phaco probe and endothelium, as well as prolonged phaco time.
5. Capsular rupture, capsular rent, or vitreous loss.
6. Loss of nucleus or nuclear fragments.
7. Iris trauma.
8. Postoperative inflammation.
9. CME.

Pertinent History

In addition to the usual ophthalmic history, surgeons should pay particular attention to the following:

1. Advanced age is correlated with hardness of the nucleus.
2. History of complications during cataract extraction in the fellow eye.
3. Vitrectomy, especially with silicone oil.
4. History of narrow angles, prior laser iridotomy, or phacomorphic glaucoma.
5. Miotic use.
6. Unstable refraction with myopic shift.
7. Need for visualization of the posterior pole for follow-up and treatment of posterior segment diseases (eg, AMD).

Clinical Evaluation

The preoperative evaluation should include a comprehensive eye examination, with consideration of the following points, depending on the specific pathology:

1. Evaluate the brow of the patient. In a case of prominent brows, consider a temporal approach for easier access.
2. Examine the endothelium for evidence of guttata or Fuchs' corneal dystrophy, because of the increased risk of corneal decompensation from prolonged phacoemulsification time, increased phacoemulsification power, and the decreased safety zone between the corneal endothelium and the phacoemulsification probe.
3. Evaluate the anterior chamber depth due to the increased diameter of the crystalline lens.
4. Perform gonioscopy to evaluate for narrow angles or iris bombé. Assess the need for laser iridotomy prior to cataract extraction if the angles are occludable (ie, phacomorphic angle-closure glaucoma).
5. Observe the degree of pupillary dilation to ensure easy access to the large lens.
6. Evaluate for signs of capsular or zonular instability (eg, trauma or pseudoexfoliation).
7. Note anterior or posterior synechiae (eg, phacomorphic glaucoma, phacolytic glaucoma with inflammation).
8. Evaluate lens color and density since intensity of brunescence correlates well with the lens hardness.
9. Perform a B-scan if there is no view of posterior fundus.

STRATEGIES TO MAXIMIZE OUTCOMES

1. To maximize patient satisfaction and promote realistic expectations, discuss any specific risks and complications of cataract surgery that are relevant to your patient. Emphasize reasonable expectations for visual outcome and other ben-

efits of surgery, the postoperative course, possibly prolonged healing time, the risk of capsular rupture and associated complications, and the risk of an AC IOL implant or possible retinal pathology not visualized at B-scan.

2. Consider laser iridotomy prior to cataract extraction if angles are occludable (ie, phacomorphic angle-closure glaucoma).

3 Discontinue any miotic agent at least 3 days prior to surgery. Phosphylene iodide should be discontinued 2 weeks before surgery.

4. Consider cyclopentolate 1% or scopolamine 0.25% one to two drops bid 2 to 3 days prior to surgery to maximize pupil dilation.

5. After consultation with the patient's internist, stop aspirin, oral NSAIDs, and other anticoagulants (such as ginkgo biloba) 10 days prior to surgery due to risk of iris bleeding, particularly if extensive iris manipulation is anticipated.

6. These patients are at high risk of surgical complications with development of CME and should receive prophylactic antiinflammatory medications.

PERIOPERATIVE CONSIDERATIONS AND MANEUVERS

Immediate Preoperative Medications

Maximize preoperative pupillary dilation with the following medications: phenylephrine 2.5% to 10%, tropicamide 1% or cyclopentolate 0.5% to 1%, and flurbiprofen 0.03% or ketorolac tromethamine 0.5% every 5 minutes x 3, starting 1 hour prior to surgery.

Anesthesia Considerations

We recommend local anesthesia in these cases. Topical or intracameral anesthesia is not our first choice due to the prolonged surgical time and greater risk of intraoperative complications. Because local anesthesia can increase retrobulbar pressure, ocular compression (with digital massage or a device such as a Honan balloon or Super-Pinky) is advocated.

Wound Construction

In order to prevent a thermal burn, consider a short scleral tunnel, which is more resistant to phaco thermal damage than a clear corneal incision. A slightly wider tunnel will permit egress of fluid around the phaco probe, which may lessen the chance of thermal injury to the wound.

Consider a temporal incision, especially if the patient has a prominent brow. This approach minimizes vertical angulation of the phaco probe, which can compress the phaco sleeve against the anterior lip of the wound, causing occlusion of cooling solution through the sleeve and resultant thermal damage.

Viscoelastic Considerations

Use generous amounts of a viscodispersive viscoelastic with high coatability (< 1 million Daltons [Viscoat]) to protect the corneal endothelium from mechanical trauma and to absorb the prolonged phacoemulsification energy. Consider using the "soft shell viscoelastic technique" described by Dr. S. Arshinoff.[2] Inject a small amount of viscodispersive viscoelastic first to coat the endothelium. Then, inject a second, high molecular weight, highly cohesive viscoelastic (ProVisc, Healon, Healon GV, or Amvisc Plus) just above the lens capsule to push the first viscoelastic against the endothelium and to maintain the anterior chamber.

Pupillary Considerations

A well-dilated pupil is essential, as the brunescent crystalline lens can be very large and the capsulorrhexis is challenging in these cases. If the pupil is still small after pharmacologic dilation, additional pupillary dilation may be necessary (see Chapter 3).

Capsulorrhexis and Other Capsular Considerations

In general, the red reflex is suboptimal in these patients but is usually sufficient to perform a capsulorrhexis. Rarely, anterior capsular staining or external transillumination with a vitreoretinal fiberoptic light probe held at the limbus may be necessary for capsular visualization (see Chapter 10).

Avoid a large capsulorrhexis because these capsules are friable and because there is a higher risk of radialization due to increased intracapsular pressure from the distended cataractous lens. Maintain sufficient viscoelastic in the anterior chamber to help control the direction of the rhexis, to tamponade nuclear prolapse, and to maintain anterior chamber depth. If necessary, the capsulorrhexis can be enlarged after placement of the IOL and before final removal of viscoelastic material.

Hydrodissection

Perform gentle, low-volume hydrodissection to avoid rupturing the friable capsule, which is already stretched due to the large nucleus. A fluid wave may not always be visible due to the lens opacity. Hydrodissection should be pursued carefully until the nucleus rotates freely. In general, hard nuclei are difficult to rotate because of corticocapsular adhesions. These may require multiple attempts at hydrodissection before phacoemulsification should be initiated.

Avoid hydrodelineation because the lens fibers do not cleave well to form an epinuclear shell and because the increased intracapsular volume can rupture the bag.

Phacoemulsification

1. Handpiece. If you are using a standard phacoemulsification tip, a 45-degree beveled tip provides better cutting for dense nuclei. There are some specialized handpiece accessories that can help reduce complications related to phacoemulsification of the hard nucleus. Alcon offers the Mackool system, with its Turbosonics Mackool microtip and two-part Mackool irrigation sleeve, to reduce thermal damage to the incision. In this system, the phaco tip is surrounded by a rigid polymer sleeve. The inner sleeve provides additional thermal protection of the cornea and scleral tissue. The rigid outer sleeve reduces friction between the tip and sleeve and maintains irrigation flow when the infusion sleeve is compressed. Alcon has also recently released the Kelman Flared Mackool ABS Tip (Alcon, Fort Worth, Tex and Richard J. Mackool, MD), which allows efficient nuclear sculpting due to its wider tip while using higher vacuum and flow settings.[3]

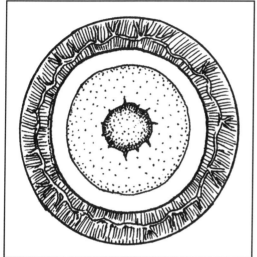

Figure 9-1. For hard nuclei, sculpting a deep central zone first will assist in nuclear cataract disassembly, regardless of the phaco technique used.

2. Settings. We recommend the use of a higher flow rate (aspiration) to increase cooling at the incision site and maintain anterior chamber depth. High power (100%) may be required to minimize lens movement during nuclear sculpting.

3. Techniques. Sculpting or chopping techniques can both be effective for removing hard, dense cataracts.[4] However, phaco-chop techniques use significantly less energy than phaco fracture methods.[5,6] With either method, it is essential to create a central area in which to emulsify nuclear fragments (Figure 9-1). Removal of the nucleus is facilitated by creating small, multiple lens pieces that are then easily emulsified and aspirated. Furthermore, using the bevel-down phaco (phaco-drill) method may further reduce energy transfer to the corneal endothelium.[7]

Cortical Aspiration

Often, there is scant cortical material remaining after removal of a dense nucleus. Thorough aspiration will help reduce postoperative inflammation without further compromise of a stressed corneal endothelium.

IOL Implantation

There are no contraindications to any of the available IOL implant materials. If a capsule-supported IOL is not possible, both sutured posterior chamber IOLs (PCIOLs) and open-loop anterior chamber IOLs (ACIOLs) have good corneal safety records. The choice of lens should depend upon the surgeon's experience.

Immediate Postoperative Medications

Use a subconjunctival injection of dexamethisone 20 to 40 mg immediately following cataract surgery to minimize postoperative inflammation.

RELEVANT POSTOPERATIVE ISSUES

Complications

1. Prolonged corneal edema. This complication can severely reduce vision for several days or weeks after surgery, but it is usually temporary and resolves after intensive topical steroid treatment. Patients with compromised corneal endothelia are at greater risk of irreversible corneal decompensation (see Chapter 2). The likelihood of corneal decompensation increases with the degree of corneal endothelial insult during surgery.

2. Inflammation due to increased phaco energy. This can be either short-term or chronic and should be treated with a postoperative steroid course accordingly.

3. Wound leak due to thermal damage. May be treated with aqueous suppressants, pressure patching, bandage contact lens, and wound revision if necessary.

4. Wound-burn associated astigmatism. Significant thermal damage to the incision may cause tissue contraction, resulting in several diopters of astigmatism. Depending on the degree of injury, this astigmatism may not regress and may require additional surgical treatment.

5. CME due to prolonged phaco time and postoperative inflammation (see Appendix C).

Postoperative Medications

1. Topical steroids. If there is extensive corneal edema, consider intensive treatment with a topical steroid (eg, prednisolone acetate 1% one to two drops every 1 to 2 hours). Also consider NSAIDs (eg, ketorolac 0.5% [Acular] or diclofenac 0.1% [Voltaren]). However, use NSAIDs sparingly in cases of corneal epithelial compromise, since there have been reports of corneal epithelial toxicity with these medications.

2. Treat IOP above 21 mmHg for patients with any corneal endothelial compromise. Avoid dorzolamide due to its potential adverse effect on the corneal endothelium.

Follow-Up

1. More frequent follow-up visits should be considered if the patient has extensive corneal edema, wound leak, intraocular inflammation, or IOP spikes.

2. If using high-dose steroids, more frequent visits are necessary to monitor the IOP.

WHEN TO CONSIDER ALTERNATIVE PROCEDURES

1. Prominent brow and deepset eye. Consider ECCE.

2. Corneal endothelial compromise. In patients with clinical evidence of corneal edema or guttata, a preoperative central corneal thickness of greater than 650 microns by corneal pachymetry may indicate the need for combined cataract surgery and penetrating keratoplasty.

3. Previous vitrectomy. Consider ECCE due to increased lens-iris diaphragm instability in order to decrease risks of zonular and capsular complications with an already friable capsule.

4. Pseudoexfoliation with capsular or zonular instability. Consider ECCE.

5. Advanced brunescent cataract. Consider ECCE depending upon phaco skill level and availability of appropriate accessory equipment.

KEY POINTS

1. Protect the corneal endothelium with viscoelastic and careful instrumentation.

2. Control the capsulorrhexis size.

3. Perform gentle hydrodissection.

4. Monitor phaco energy and effects (thermal wound damage).

5. During nuclear disassembly, maintain small fragments.

6. Use prophylactic medications for CME (see Appendix C).

REFERENCES

1. Dada T, Sharma, N, Vajpayee RB, et al. Conversion from phacoemulsification to extra-capsular cataract extraction: incidence, risk factors, and visual outcomes. *J Cataract Refract Surg.* 1998;24(11):1521-1524.

2. Arshinoff SA. Dispersive-cohesive viscoelastic soft shell technique. *J Cataract Refract Surg.* 1999;25(2):167-173.

3. Bissen-Miyajima H, Shimmura S, Tsubota K. Thermal effect on corneal incisions with different phacoemulsification ultrasonic tips. *J Cataract Refract Surg.* 1999;25(1):60-64.

4. Vasavada A, Singh R. Step-by-step chop in situ and separation of very dense cataracts. *J Cataract Refract Surg.* 1998;24(2):156-159.

5. Pirazzoli G, D'Eliseo D, Ziosi M, et al. Effects of phacoemulsification time on the corneal endothelium using phacofracture and phaco chop techniques. *J Cataract Refract Surg.* 1996;22(7):967-969.

6. DeBry P, Olson RJ, Crandall AS. Comparison of energy required for phaco-chop and divide and conquer phacoemulsification. *J Cataract Refract Surg.* 1998;24(5):689-692.

7. Joo CK, Kim YH. Phacoemulsification with a bevel-down phaco tip: phaco-drill. *J Cataract Refract Surg.* 1997;23(8):1149-1152.

10

THE WHITE CATARACT

Richard J. Maw, MD
Roberto Pineda II, MD

RELEVANT PREOPERATIVE ISSUES

Clinical Settings

Terms such as opaque, mature, hypermature, advanced, and intumescent have been used to describe white cataracts. Regardless of terminology, every surgeon who has encountered a white cataract knows the special challenge that these cases present. White cataracts are most often seen in the context of sub-optimal or delayed medical care, and are sometimes associated with extensive ultraviolet exposure, uveitis, ocular trauma, or diabetes. Achievement of a continuous, curvilinear capsulorrhexis (CCC) is especially difficult. This is due to several factors: lack of a red reflex, difficulty controlling the capsulorrhexis due to increased intracapsular/intralenticular pressure, problems recognizing radial tears, and a "milky" cortex obscuring the surgeon's view. The use of dyes to stain the anterior capsule, along with several other special maneuvers greatly enhance the surgeon's chance for a successful surgery. These techniques will be described in this chapter.

Risks and Complications

Patients with a white cataract may have greater incidences of the following complications:

1. Incomplete capsulorrhexis (5% to 28.3%).[1,2]
2. Corneal edema (5.7% to 26%).[1,2]
3. IOL decentration (20%).[1]
4. Capsular bag contraction (12%).[1]
5. Elevated IOP greater than 26 mmHg (5%).[1]
6. Intraoperative miosis (3.3%).[2]
7. Posterior capsular tear (1.9%).[2]
8. Conversion to manual ECCE (1.9%).[2]
9. Persistent iritis (0.9%).[2]

10. Residual cortex.

11. Vitreous loss.

12. Average endothelial cell loss of 18% at 6 months.[1]

Pertinent History

In addition to the usual ophthalmic history, surgeons should pay particular attention to the following:

1. Past ocular trauma.

2. Retinal pathology.

3. Glaucoma.

4. Uveitis.

5. Diabetes.

6. Previous surgery (eg, PPV, gas injection, etc).

Clinical Evaluation

The preoperative evaluation should include a comprehensive eye examination, with consideration of the following points, depending on the specific pathology:

1. Visual acuity will likely be hand motion or light perception with projection. Visual acuity of light perception without projection suggests a poor prognosis due to advanced retinal and/or optic nerve pathology.

2. Examination for a relative afferent pupillary defect (RAPD) must be performed. A patient with a normal functioning optic nerve will not have an afferent pupillary defect in the presence of a white cataract.

3. Search for evidence of a compromised corneal endothelium such as guttata or corneal edema. Consider specular microscopy and pachymetry, since some dyes used to stain the anterior capsule can stress the corneal endothelium.

4. Identify signs of uveitis, including posterior synechiae, old keratic precipitates (KP), and rubeosis irides.

5. Signs of phacodonesis are best observed by asking the patient to move the eyes briefly at the slit lamp.

6. Increased intracapsular/intralenticular pressure can frequently be detected at the slit lamp by an increased convexity of the central, anterior lens.[3]

7. IOL calculations may be erroneous due to difficulty obtaining axial length and keratometry measurements in these nonfixating eyes. Measurements should be compared to the fellow eye to confirm their accuracy.

8. A B-scan is required to rule out retinal detachment and intraocular masses.

STRATEGIES TO MAXIMIZE OUTCOMES

1. To maximize patient satisfaction and promote realistic expectations, discuss any specific risks and complications of cataract surgery listed on the previous page that are relevant to your patient. Also discuss reasonable expectations for

visual outcome given the uncertainty of visual potential.

2. In the presence of strabismus, the patient must be warned about the possibility of postoperative diplopia and the possible need for strabismus surgery at a later date.

3. Determine the ability of the iris to dilate. If there is poor pupillary dilation, plan to stretch the pupil before the capsulorrhexis is attempted (see Chapter 3).

4. Consider pretreatment with topical steroids before surgery, due to a higher risk of severe postoperative inflammation (eg, prednisolone acetate qid for 3 days prior to surgery).

5. The surgeon should be ready to convert to a manual ECCE if the planned phacoemulsification becomes compromised.

PERIOPERATIVE CONSIDERATIONS AND TECHNIQUES

Immediate Preoperative Medications

Use a routine antibiotic and dilation regimen. If there is poor dilation of the pupil, 10% phenylephrine (use carefully for patients with cardiac problems) and repeated application of tropicamide 1% can augment dilation.

Anesthesia Considerations

Local anesthesia is strongly recommended. Adequate akinesia is necessary during the capsulorrhexis, and adequate anesthesia is necessary if the case is converted to a manual ECCE.

Wound Construction

A short, limbal scleral tunnel is recommended due to the possibility of converting to a manual ECCE or ICCE.

Viscoelastic Considerations

Several different viscoelastics can be employed. If the corneal endothelium is not compromised, it is reasonable to use a high molecular weight viscoelastic alone (eg, Healon, Healon GV, or Amvisc Plus) to augment anterior chamber stability during the capsulorrhexis.

However, if the corneal endothelium is compromised, we recommend first using a viscodispersive viscoelastic (such as Viscoat) to coat the corneal endothelium. This is followed by aspiration of Viscoat from the anterior chamber while leaving a protective coating of Viscoat on the corneal endothelium. An air bubble may be placed into the anterior chamber, the capsular dye placed, and the capsulorrhexis performed as described below.

Pupillary Considerations

A small pupil can be managed in a variety of ways: sector iridectomy, circumferential microsphincterotomies, iris hooks, and pupil stretching to provide greater pupillary dilation (see Chapter 3).

Capsulorrhexis and Other Capsular Considerations

As mentioned earlier, creation of a capsulorrhexis is the most important and most difficult part of phacoemulsification in the white cataract. The absence of a red reflex, increased intracapsular pressure, dispersion of liquid milky cortex, difficulty controlling the capsulorrhexis, and trouble recognizing radial tears all combine to make achieving a capsulorrhexis a significant challenge. Dimming the operating room lights, a good focus with high magnification, frequent rewetting of the cornea, and a vitreoretinal fiberoptic light probe held outside the eye against the limbus for coaxial illumination are all helpful in successfully completing the capsulorrhexis.

However, staining of the anterior capsule is the most useful adjunct when performing a capsulorrhexis in the absence of a good red reflex. Multiple dyes have been used for this purpose, including indocyanine green (ICG [Bausch & Lomb, St. Louis, Mo]) 0.5%, trypan blue 0.1% (Vision Blue [Dutch Ophthalmic Research Corp, or DORC, Kingston, NH]), fluorescein 2% (Minims [Akorn Inc, Lincolnshire, Ill]), gentian violet, and methylene blue.[4-8] ICG has been reported to provide the best staining and easiest recognition of the anterior capsule.[4,7] Trypan blue and fluorescein have also been reported to work well in several studies.[4-6] However, gentian violet and methylene blue may be associated with an increased incidence of corneal edema;[6,8] and fluorescein has been reported to diffuse into the viscoelastic, stain the corneal endothelium, and leak into the vitreous cavity.[4] The authors have used ICG, trypan blue, and fluorescein with excellent results, although we do agree that ICG provides slightly better capsular visualization than the other two. ICG is made as follows: 25 mg is dissolved in 0.5 mL[l] of aqueous solvent (provided with the ICG) and is then mixed with 4.5 mL[l] of a balanced salt solution.

Our technique is currently as follows: make a small paracentesis just large enough for the cannula. Fill the anterior chamber completely with air, and seal the paracentesis with viscoelastic. If dye is dripping out of the cannula when it is introduced into the eye, capillary action will draw the dye onto the iris and corneal endothelium, thereby obscuring the view. Consequently, we "seed" the end of the cannula with air to prevent this capillary action. Next, place the cannula into the anterior chamber and inject the dye (from a tuberculin syringe) so that one or two microdroplets fall onto the center of the anterior capsule (Figure 10-1). Then, use the barrel of the cannula to paint or brush the capsule with the dye.

Viscoelastic is then injected into the anterior chamber such that the air bubble egresses through the paracentesis. A scleral tunnel incision is then constructed. Because there may be high intracapsular pressure, it is important to use the cystotome to make a small, initial tear in the center of the anterior capsule. Take a moment here to observe what happens. If high intracapsular pressure causes a radial tear in the capsule, a capsulorrhexis can be started from this tear. If the dye or milky cortex obscures the view, use irrigation and aspiration to remove it and reintroduce new viscoelastic. The dark dye, which stains the posterior surface of the anterior capsule, will show distinctly against the white cataract. Consequently, a capsulorrhexis can usually be achieved with excellent visibility of the capsular tears' leading edge (Figure 10-2).

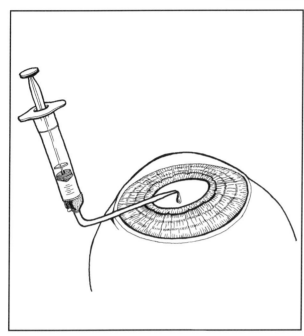

Figure 10-1. Capsular staining with air in the anterior chamber. Hold the cannula above the central capsule. Otherwise the dye has a tendency to migrate along the cannula into the angle, heavily staining the iris and other ocular structures. The drop of dye can then be painted onto the anterior capsular surface.

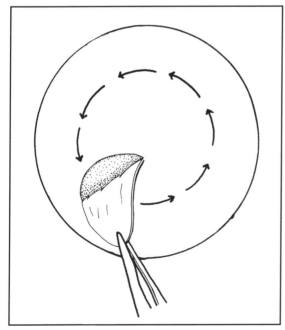

Figure 10-2. Although not obvious after anterior capsule staining, once the capsulorrhexis is initiated, the tinted capsule contrasts easily with the underlying white cataract.

Hydrodissection

Assuming a capsulorrhexis has been achieved, proceed with routine gentle hydrodissection. Inject balanced salt solution at multiple locations since a fluid wave cannot be seen. Test the lens for mobility.

Phacoemulsification

Be prepared to encounter the full range of nuclear hardness. If the nucleus is soft, sometimes the entire lens can be removed with just irrigation and aspiration. However, it is also possible to encounter nuclei of 4+ to 5+ hardness. In such cases, using a high cavitation tip such as the Kelman tip on the Alcon system 20,000 Legacy can be helpful.

Cortical Aspiration

Frequently no cortical clean-up is needed. When cortical clean-up is required, proceed with routine irrigation and aspiration.

IOL Implantation

If the capsular bag is intact, a foldable IOL implant can be placed in the bag. If the lens cannot be placed in the bag, a one-piece PMMA lens with a 6.0 mm or larger optic should be used to minimize problems due to decentration.

RELEVANT POSTOPERATIVE ISSUES

Complications

1. Thus far, no increase in corneal edema has been described from the use of ICG, fluorescein, and trypan blue.[4-7] Gentian violet and methylene blue may have toxic effects.[6,8]

2. Diplopia from strabismus may continue to improve for months if the strabismus was due to sensory deprivation from the white cataract. Therefore, one should not proceed with strabismus surgery for at least 3 months after cataract surgery (and documentation of stable measurements).

Postoperative Medications

1. Consider intensive treatment with a topical steroid (prednisolone acetate 1% one to two drops every 1 to 2 hours) if extensive iris manipulation.

2. Consider NSAIDs (eg, ketorolac 0.5% [Acular] or diclofenac 0.1% [Voltaren]).

Follow-Up

1. More frequent follow-up is required if there were complications during surgery. Inflammation and IOP should be well-controlled.

2. A full, dilated fundus examination should be performed shortly after surgery since it was not possible before surgery. Prompt treatment of any pathology (eg, retinal holes, diabetic retinopathy, etc) should be initiated.

WHEN TO CONSIDER ALTERNATIVE PROCEDURES

1. Preoperative presence of an RAPD or visual acuity of light perception without projection suggests advanced retinal and/or optic nerve pathology that will probably limit visual acuity. Reconsider need for cataract surgery.

2. Previous history of pars plana vitrectomy (especially in the presence of inflammation) may be a sign that the posterior capsule is compromised, and the surgeon may opt for a planned, manual ECCE.

3. If the IOP is poorly controlled, consider a two-stage combined procedure (cataract removal, IOL implantation, and trabeculectomy). One option is as follows: perform phacoemulsification using a temporal approach, then intraoperatively examine the optic nerve for signs of glaucomatous damage. If significant glaucomatous damage is noted, proceed with trabeculectomy in the superior quadrant.

4. If there is significant phacodonesis, plan for a manual ECCE or ICCE with a closed-loop ACIOL, or a scleral suture-fixated PCIOL, depending on the surgeon's experience. Similarly, if there is a history of trauma to the eye, the surgeon may opt for a planned, manual ECCE and thereby avoid inadvertent zonular rupture.

5. If there is a prior history of pars plana vitrectomy, the surgeon may opt for a planned, manual ECCE. The reasons are two-fold: first, there may be a pre-existing posterior capsular tear induced during the vitrectomy. Second, the lack of posterior vitreal support for the crystalline lens adds to the already increased chance of complications during phacoemulsification.

KEY POINTS

1. A B-scan is required preoperatively to rule out retinal detachment and intraocular masses.

2. The use of dye to stain the anterior capsule provides excellent visibility of the leading edge of the capsulorrhexis.

3. ICG provides the best visibility of the known dyes. Trypan blue and fluorescein also work well.

4. Local anesthesia is preferable to topical anesthesia.

5. A scleral tunnel incision is recommended in case of likely conversion to a manual ECCE.

6. A planned, manual ECCE is recommended for a history of significant trauma, previous pars plana vitrectomy, phacodonesis, or iridonesis.

7. An immediate dilated postoperative examination is essential.

8. If a capsulorrhexis is accomplished, the success rate of phacoemulsification for white cataracts is similar to that of routine cataract surgery.

COMMERCIAL DYE INFORMATION

Trypan Blue Dye

Sold as a box of 10 sterile, premixed individual vials for approximately $100 US. The US Food and Drug Administration approval is currently pending. It is available outside of the United States, including Canada and Europe (DORC, 800-75-DUTCH).

ICG Dye

Sold in packages of six applications for $330 US. Each application consists of two vials: one containing 25 mg of lyophilized ICG powder and a second containing 0.5 cc of diluent. The ICG powder is dissolved in the diluent, and the resulting solution is then mixed with 4.5 cc of sterile balanced salt solution-plus for a final concentration of 0.5% ICG. Use a low-volume filtering disc such as Millipore filters (Millipore, Bedford, Mass) to filter the final solution (ACORN, 800-535-7155).

Fluorescein 2% Dye

Sold in single sterile, prepackaged droperettes. Can be used directly intracamerally without dilution. Alcon and Ciba Vison have discontinued manufacturing. Bausch & Lomb makes a 0.25% in a 5 mL bottle (800-323-0000).

REFERENCES

1. Vasavada A, Singh R, Desai J. Phacoemulsification of white mature cataracts. *J Cataract Refract Surg*. 1998;24(2):270-7.

2. Chakrabarti A, Sing S, Krishnadas R. Phacoemulsification in eyes with white cataract. *J Cataract Refract Surg*. 2000;26(7):1041-1047.

3. Surendra B. Different faces of a white cataract: A Phaco Surgeon's Perspective. *Aust N Z J Ophthalmol*. 1990;27:53-56.

4. Pandey S, Werner L, Escobar-Gomez M, et al. Dye enhanced cataract surgery part 1: anterior capsule staining for capsulorrhexis in advanced/white cataract. *J Cataract Refract Surg*. 2000;26(7):1052-1059.

5. Gotzaridis E, Ayliffe W. Fluorescein dye improves visualization during capsulorrhexis in mature cataracts. *J Cataract Refract Surg*. 1999;25(11):1423.

6. Melles G, de Waard P, Pameyer J, et al. Trypan blue capsule staining to visualize the capsulorrhexis in cataract surgery. *J Cataract Refract Surg*. 1999;25(1):7-9

7. Horiguchi M, Miyake K, Ohta I, et al. Staining of the lens capsule for circular continuous capsulorrhexis in eyes with white cataract. *Arch Ophthalmol*. 1998;116(4):535-537.

8. Unlu K, Askunger A, Soker S, et al. Gentian violet staining for the anterior capsule. *J Cataract Refract Surg*. 2000;26(8):1228-1232.

9. Chylack L, Leke M, Sperduto R. Lens opacities classification system. *Arch Ophthalmol*. ·1998;106:330-334.

10. Gimbel H, Willerscheidt A. What to do with a limited view: the intumescent cataract. *J Cataract Refract Surg*. 1993;19:657-661.

THE TRAUMATIC CATARACT

Eugene S. Lit, MD
Victor L. Perez, MD
Susannah G. Rowe, MD, MPH
Roberto Pineda II, MD

RELEVANT PREOPERATIVE ISSUES

Clinical Settings

In general, the majority of traumatic cataracts can be safely removed with posterior chamber IOLs and improvement in visual acuity.[1] A complication rate of 15% in traumatic cataracts has been reported.[1] Traumatic cataracts occur most often in younger patients. They can occur in blunt trauma, penetrating or perforating injury with either direct or indirect involvement of the lens, and rarely with electrocution. Traumatic cataracts can occur from hours to years after the injury and are often associated with other complications, such as zonular or capsular rupture, traumatic uveitis, glaucoma, hyphema, and other numerous ocular injuries. The indications for removal of a traumatic cataract can be acute, semiacute, or elective. This chapter concentrates on the elective removal of traumatic cataracts, with select references to acute and subacute settings.

Acute

- In general, primary cataract extraction is performed only if there is a high suspicion of worsening lens-related inflammation, loss of fragments into the posterior segment, or significant risk of lens particle glaucoma from a highly disrupted lens capsule. In the acute setting, it is difficult to obtain accurate measurements for IOL calculations. This chapter will cover IOL estimations in this setting (see Appendix A).

Semiacute

- Occasionally, the crystalline lens may need to be removed early in the postoperative course due to persistent inflammation, phacoanaphylactic/phacoantigenic uveitis, or lens particle glaucoma. The development of phacoanaphylactic/phacoantigenic uveitis is an absolute indication for immediate cataract extraction.

Elective

- Elective cataract extraction is preferred, as it permits more accurate measurements for IOL power calculations. In addition, some small traumatic cataracts do not progress. If the capsule defect heals before lens hydration reaches the visual axis, then removal of the lens can sometimes be avoided. Finally, waiting to perform cataract surgery ensures that any open globe wounds are more stable. Cataracts arising from blunt trauma, but without perforating trauma, usually fall into the elective category.

Risks and Complications

Patients with a traumatic cataract may have greater incidences of the following complications:

1. Unanticipated postoperative refractive error (due to inaccurate biometric measurements for IOL calculation and lens malposition).

2. Prolonged postoperative corneal edema, especially in the setting of previous endothelial cell damage (trauma, glaucoma, or hyphema).

3. Exuberant postoperative inflammation.

4. Prolonged postoperative increase in IOP. These patients have multiple risk factors for traumatic glaucoma.

5. Hyphema.

6. IOL dislocation/subluxation with diplopia and other optical aberrations.

7. Higher incidence of posterior capsular opacification for younger patients.[2]

8. Need for additional surgeries (IOL exchange, removal, etc).

9. Increased risk of posterior capsular rupture and associated complications (unstable capsule or occult tears).

10. Vitreous loss.

11. Nuclear fragment loss through posterior capsular breaks, zonular breaks.

12. Increased risk of retinal detachment.

13. CME (see Appendix C).

Pertinent History

In addition to the usual ophthalmic history, surgeons should pay particular attention to the following:

1. Pretrauma ocular conditions (refractive error, glaucoma, diabetic retinopathy, etc).

2. Post-traumatic ocular complications (history of traumatic glaucoma, hypotony, severe inflammation, hyphema, retinal detachment, or optic neuropathy).

3. Mechanism of injury.

4. History of intraocular foreign body (IOFB), especially metallic.[3]

5. Ophthalmic surgical and medical interventions.

6. History of associated nonocular trauma.

7. Date of injury and surgical repair.

8. Ocular medications.

9. Induced myopia/astigmatism or monocular diplopia. A subluxed crystalline lens may cause these symptoms from the peripheral lenticular edge effect.

Clinical Evaluation

The preoperative evaluation should include a comprehensive eye examination, with consideration of the following points, depending on the specific pathology:

1. Careful refraction of the fellow eye and of the injured eye whenever possible.

2. Examination for a RAPD must be performed to assess for traumatic optic neuropathy. A patient with a normal functioning optic nerve will not have an afferent pupillary defect even in the presence of an opaque cataract.

3. Evaluate for persistent corneal edema, scarring, severe astigmatism, corneal endothelial blood staining, signs of endothelial decompensation (guttata, pigment, or edema), and corneal sutures from previous laceration repair. Consider specular microscopy and pachymetry if corneal endothelial decompensation is suspected, since some dyes used to stain the anterior capsule can stress the corneal endothelium.

4. Persistent inflammation (traumatic or phacoantigenic), persistent microhyphema, vitreous in the anterior segment and vitreous in the wound.

5. Gonioscopy: Evaluate angle for recession or fibrosis, foamy macrophages, anterior synechiae, iridodialysis, or cyclodialysis.

6. Measure maximal pupillary dilation. Note any iridocapsular synechiae.

7. Assess for the presence of traumatic iris deformities, iridocorneal adhesions, posterior synechiae, or iridodonesis with gonioscopy.

8. Dilated slit lamp examination is the best method for examining the crystalline lens after trauma. Look carefully for signs of capsular rupture. Note the presence and location of a fibrotic anterior capsular plaque. Subtle signs of zonular instability, including lens dislocation, iridodonesis, or phacodonesis, can be elicited if the patient makes several rapid eye movements at the slit lamp. Retroillumination also can be helpful in evaluating subtle lens subluxation and identifying areas of compromised zonules.

9. Evaluate the adequacy of the red reflex for capsulorrhexis.

10. Careful examination of the vitreous body and posterior segment (macula, retina, and optic nerve) should be performed to assess the integrity of vital essential structures.

11. *If the posterior segment cannot be clearly visualized, a B-scan is required to rule out a retinal detachment or an x-ray to rule out an IOFB.*

12. B-scan or immersion ultrasound biomicroscopy can be helpful in detecting posterior capsular tears.

13. If there is a history of an IOFB, or if an IOFB is present, perform an electroretinogram (ERG) to assess retinal function and signs of retinal toxicity.

14. In nonfixating eyes, IOL calculations may be erroneous due to difficulty obtaining axial length and keratometry measurements in these nonfixating eyes. Measurements should be compared to the fellow eye to confirm their accuracy.

15. If cataract surgery is performed at the time of initial repair, use the axial length and keratometry measurements of the uninvolved eye if the patient has a history of identical vision in both eyes. Do not perform A-scan/B-scan on an open globe.

STRATEGIES TO MAXIMIZE OUTCOMES

1. To maximize patient satisfaction and promote realistic expectations, discuss any specific risks and complications of cataract surgery listed that are relevant to your patient. Also, discuss reasonable expectations for visual outcome given the uncertainty of the visual potential. Be sure to consult the patient about other possible procedures, including aphakia, sutured IOL, and vitrectomy.

2. Defer elective cataract surgery until the eye has stabilized from the trauma and any surgical repairs.

3. If there is poor pupillary dilation, plan to stretch the pupil before the capsulorrhexis is attempted (see Chapter 3). Operating through a small pupil will increase your risk of complications.

4. Consider pretreatment with topical steroids before surgery due to a higher risk of severe postoperative inflammation (ie, prednisolone acetate qid for 3 days prior to surgery).

5. Prepare to convert to a manual ECCE if the planned phacoemulsification becomes compromised.

6. Preoperatively, use topical NSAIDs and steroids for CME prophylaxis (see Appendix C).

IOL Considerations

1. Plan to balance the refraction in the fellow eye to within 2 to 3 D. Always err on the myopic side.

2. A 6.0-mm optic IOL allows an extra margin of safety if the IOL becomes mildly decentered. Ideally, the overall IOL diameter should be 13 mm, and it should be no smaller than 12.

3. PMMA haptics are often preferred since they are stiffer and may help prevent capsular contraction and IOL decentration. We have used the following IOLs with good results: foldable one-piece acrylic, foldable acrylic with PMMA haptics, and one-piece PMMA. We do not recommend silicone IOLs unless there is no involvement of the posterior segment.

4. Heparin surface-modified and acrylic IOLs have been postulated to minimize corneal edema, anterior chamber reaction, formation of synechiae, and IOL

deposits. However, over the long-term, the lower incidence of these events has not yet been demonstrated to be statistically significant.

5. Silicone IOLs are not a good choice if the patient is likely to undergo an air/fluid exchange (due to condensation),[8] or to require a vitreous substitute such as silicone oil (due to irreversible silicone oil adhesion to the silicone IOL).[4]

6. Many surgeons are uncomfortable with placing an ACIOL in younger patients due to the risk of glaucoma. A sutured IOL should be considered in cases of inadequate capsular support. If there is significant traumatic injury to the trabecular meshwork, an ACIOL should probably be avoided. In elderly patients with no evidence of trabecular meshwork damage, ACIOLs may be acceptable.

PERIOPERATIVE CONSIDERATIONS AND TECHNIQUES

Immediate Preoperative Medications

Use a routine antibiotic and dilation regimen. If there is poor dilation of the pupil, 10% phenylephrine and repeated application of cyclopentolate 1% or tropicamide 0.5% to 1% can augment dilation. Be sure you are aware of the patient's medical condition before you administer these drugs.

Anesthesia Considerations

Local anesthesia is strongly recommended. Adequate akinesia is necessary during the capsulorrhexis, and adequate anesthesia is necessary if the case is converted to a manual ECCE. Topical and intracameral anesthesia should be avoided in cases of phacodonesis and zonular dialysis.

Avoid stressing the zonules by overpressuring the eye at the start of surgery. For this reason, it is best to avoid ocular compression of the globe after administering anesthesia (ie, avoid digital massage, Super-Pinky, or Honan balloon). For the same reason, do not inject an excessive volume of anesthetic during a peribulbar or retrobulbar injection.

Wound Construction

1. A short, limbal scleral tunnel is recommended due to the possibility of converting to a manual ECCE or ICCE.

2. Construct the incision so that the least stress will be placed on any broken zonules (ie, 180 degrees away from the area of zonular weakness). If an asymmetric corneal opacity is present, try to position the incision to maximize visualization of the anterior chamber (ie, temporal versus superior approach).

3. Clear corneal incisions should be avoided if there is significant corneal trauma or corneal endothelial cell damage.

4. If lens removal is anticipated using a vitrector alone (as with younger patients who have very soft lenses), the initial wound should be small (see Special Techniques section).

Viscoelastic Considerations

Avoid hyperinflation of the anterior chamber while injecting viscoelastic, as this can force the lens posteriorly and rupture the zonules, potentially compromising the capsule.

In the presence of a small pupil, use a high-molecular weight, highly cohesive viscoelastic (ProVisc, Healon, Healon GV, or Amvisc Plus) to facilitate dilation of the pupil and help control iris bleeding should pupil enlarging techniques be employed. If the corneal endothelium is compromised, we recommend first using a viscodispersive viscoelastic such as Viscoat, to coat the corneal endothelium. This is followed by a high molecular weight, highly cohesive viscoelastic aspiration of Viscoat from the anterior chamber which provides anterior chamber maintenance while pushing the Viscoat toward the cornea, leaving a protective coating of Viscoat on the corneal endothelium.

Pupillary Considerations

1. A small pupil secondary to synechia adhesions can occur in the traumatic cataract, especially if there was significant post-traumatic inflammation. In order to maximize pupil dilation and adequate access to the lens, any iris adhesions to the anterior capsule should be carefully lysed. This can be done with a Sinskey, Kuglen, Y-hook, or a similar fish-hook cyclodialysis type of instrument inserted through the paracentesis incision at the beginning of the procedure (see Figure 5-1). Once freed from the anterior capsule, the iris can be further dilated using iris hooks, bimanual stretching, radial iridotomy, or sphincterectomies (see Chapter 3).

2. Repair of any iris defects can be made at the time of elective cataract removal. This is usually done after removal of the cataract and placement of the IOL. The exception is usually when the patient has an iridodialysis, preventing good visualization of the cataract. The iridodialysis is then repaired.

Capsulorrhexis and Other Capsular Considerations

1. Be sure to remove any prolapsed vitreous prior to beginning the capsulorrhexis.

2. If the patient is young and an attempt is being made to first remove as much of the lens by irrigation/aspiration as possible, do not complete the capsulorrhexis immediately. A slit in the anterior capsule (which can later be used to initiate the capsulorrhexis if needed) is made, and the vitrector is passed through this. During irrigation/aspiration, if a larger opening is needed, this can be done with the vitrector.

3. Consider using techniques that limit strain on the zonules. The surface of the lens capsule can be hard to perforate with a cystotome without excessive downward force on the lens. Pinch-type forceps (eg, Kershner capsulorrhexis cystotome forceps [Rhein Medical]) have sharp tips that simultaneously grasp the capsule and initiate the tear without pressing down onto the lens. If it is difficult to complete a continuous curvilinear capsulorrhexis without stressing the zonules, consider converting to a can-opener technique capsulotomy. Should a radialization tear occur, which cannot be recovered, have a low threshold to convert to ECCE.

4. Commonly in younger patients with traumatic cataracts, a dense fibrotic anterior subcapsular plaque will develop. These plaques can greatly complicate the capsulorrhexis. *Do not* try to tear through these plaques! When performing the capsulorrhexis, start far away from the plaque and tear completely around the

plaque if at all possible. The plaque will usually lift off as a single stiff unit. If it is not possible to tear around the plaque, then tear up to the plaque and use scissors to cut through the plaque (this may be easy or difficult). Usually, an intact capsulorrhexis can be achieved (Figure 11-1).

5. If there is a poor red reflex due to a dense white cataract, consider capsular staining techniques to facilitate the capsulorrhexis (see Chapter 10).

Hydrodissection/Hydrodelineation

Keep in mind that there may be weakness or tears in the posterior capsule that have gone undetected. Aggressive hydrodissection may cause a hydraulic rupture at the point of capsular compromise, and a posterior tear can then extend peripherally. Therefore, perform gentle, low-volume hydrodissection in multiple quandrants. A fluid wave may not always be visible due to the lens opacity. Hydrodissection should be thoroughly pursued to cleave the cortical material from the capsule, thereby minimizing stress on the zonules during lens removal.

Hydrodelineation may also be useful, depending upon the density of the nucleus and the integrity of the lens-zonular complex. If there are less than 3 clock-hours of zonular dialysis and if there is no evidence of iridodonesis and phacodonesis, then hydrodelineation should probably be performed. This technique creates a small endonucleus that can be phacoemulsified more easily. Even more importantly, it creates an epinuclear shell, protecting the posterior capsule during nuclear cataract removal and allows removal of the epinuclear plate and cortex material with the least amount of trauma to the lens-zonular complex.

Phacoemulsification

Be sure to remove any vitreous from the anterior chamber before introducing the phacoemulsification probe into the eye. If you cannot be sure whether there is vitreous in the anterior chamber or not, remove as much of the lens as possible using the vitrector (see Special Techniques).

In the absence of vitreous in the anterior chamber, modified phacoemulsification techniques may be performed.

Keep the Bottle Height Low

- To minimize hyperinflation of the anterior chamber and downward stress on the zonules, minimize displacement of the lens while removing the nucleus. Standard divide-and-conquer techniques can stress the zonules; therefore, we suggest the use of a nonrotational cracking or chopping technique.

Use Sufficient Power to Minimize Lens Displacement

- Consider a high-cavitation phaco tip (eg, Kelman tip) that emulsifies nuclear material beyond the tip and thereby minimizes dragging of the lens while sculpting. This technique allows an initial groove to be formed. Without rotating the lens, a lateral and rotational motion of the phaco probe can groove the nucleus in a lateral direction.[2]

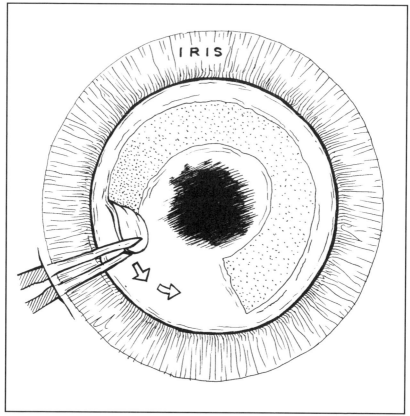

Figure 11-1. A dense fibrotic anterior capsular plaque may occur after ocular trauma. The capsulorrhexis should circumnavigate the plaque if at all possible. Otherwise, it is necessary to transect the plaque using angled Gills scissors in order to generate an intact capsulorrhexis and prevent a radial capsular tear.

Stabilize the Nucleus with a Second Instrument Through the Paracentesis Site if Lens Movement is Noted During Phacoemulsification

- One can also push the nucleus toward the phaco tip while elevating the lens slightly. If rotation is necessary, rotate using both instruments simultaneously, placed at opposite poles of the nucleus, to maximize spinning without stressing the zonules.

In younger patients, large portions of the lens may be aspirated. Using a manual irrigation/aspiration handpiece, like the Simcoe, may help maintain control. It is often useful to separate out the irrigation port to a separate line (see Relevant Postoperative Issues).

When more than 1 or 2 clock hours of the zonules are lost, the capsule may collapse easily during phacoemulsification, causing further stripping of the zonules and risking capsular dehiscence or rent. This collapse may be counteracted by reinflating the bag repeatedly with a high molecular weight viscoelastic (eg, Healon, Healon GV, or Amvisc Plus). Be prepared to repeatedly fill the capsule with viscoelastic, since the viscoelastic will be aspirated during phacoemulsification.

Cortical Aspiration

If there is an area of suspected zonular instability with an intact anterior capsulorrhexis and posterior capsule, consider placement of the IOL prior to cortical removal. Positioning one haptic in the meridian at the point of zonular instability may help support the capsular bag and zonules in this area. Do not drag the cortex centrally; it is safer to strip it tangentially (circumferentially). Apply tractional forces in the direction of any areas of zonular dehiscence rather than away from them. Injecting viscoelastic between the cortex and capsule (ie, viscodissection) sometimes aids in less traumatic cortex removal. This may also be considered at the time of hydrodissection if the capsular bag is not compromised. Using a manual irrigation/aspiration handpiece (Simcoe) may provide better control.

Keep the bottle height low to minimize hyperinflation of the AC and downward stress on the zonules.

IOL Implantation

Verify that the capsular bag is intact with sufficient zonular support, prior to placing an endocapsular or sulcus-fixated IOL. If capsular support for the IOL is uncertain, leave the trailing haptic outside the wound when first placing the lens. When there is insufficient support, it will become more obvious as the lens tilts down. With the haptic still accessible, the lens can be easily removed. If the lens appears stable, the haptic can be maneuvered into the sulcus or bag with angled MacPherson forceps.

Use an ACIOL or sutured PCIOL (depending on the surgeon's experience) when there is not sufficient zonular support for the lens. This is usually the case when there are greater than 4 clock hours of zonular dehiscence.

When placing foldable IOLs, consider folding the lens in the "taco" configuration or using an injector, such that both haptics will unfold simultaneously into the bag. This will lessen rotational traction on the zonules. Otherwise, consider dunking rather than rotating (dialing) the trailing haptic for the same reason.

If the capsular bag appears to be well-supported but there is an area of suspected zonular instability, position one haptic at the weakest point to provide regional zonular support to the capsular bag and zonules in that area. Additionally, this will help prevent prolapse of vitreous anteriorly.

Wound Closure

We recommend closing the tunnel with at least one suture, since trauma patients often require additional surgical procedures.

Special Techniques

1. Lens removal with vitrectomy. This technique should be considered when vitreous is suspected in the anterior chamber. In general, it is used in younger patients when significant portions of the very soft nucleus (or the entire lens) can be removed using irrigation and aspiration. The vitrector may be inserted through a paracentesis at the limbus or through a small opening within a scleral tunnel. For this procedure, we recommend using the 3-step settings for the pedal. This will allow the surgeon to switch instantly from aspiration to cutting when vitreous is encountered.

2. Capsular ring (see Figure 4-1). An endocapsular ring (Morcher, Germany) is placed inside the capsular bag immediately after the capsulorrhexis to keep the bag stretched throughout the procedure.[2,3,5] The rings come in three sizes (normal = 10 mm, large = 11 mm, extra-large = 12 mm). Endocapsular rings distribute any forces to the entire zonular ring, stabilizing the equator of the bag during cortical aspiration and expanding the bag to facilitate IOL implantation. The ring remains in place after surgery and helps resist capsular contraction due to metaplasia and fibrosis of the capsulorrhexis.

3. Microhooks. Capsular microhook retractors are similar to pupillary retractors.[6] These microhooks can be used in conjunction with endocapsular rings or by themselves. Four small, flexible hooks are inserted through corneal paracentesis sites to capture the capsulorrhexis edge. The hooks are then retracted gently, stretching the capsulotomy and stabilizing the lens at four points.[3] The hooks lessen rotation as well as posterior movement of the bag. They are removed at the end of the case.

4. Anterior vitrectomy. We suggest two-port vitrectomy to manage capsular ruptures with vitreous prolapse into the anterior chamber. The infusion cannula can be used separately and directed away from the capsular defect into the peripheral anterior angle. This will lessen turbulence at the cutter tip and reduce hydration of the vitreous, thereby lowering the risk of capsular tear extension. The vitrector should be used with a high cutting rate and low vacuum/aspiration flow rates (ie, cut rate = 400 cuts/min, vacuum = 100 mm Hg, aspiration = 5 cc/min). Vitrectomy should be carried out with slow and circumferential movements, beginning anteriorly and moving toward the capsular bag, and close to the area of the rupture. Distortion of the pupillary margin should alert the surgeon to persistent vitreous material in the anterior chamber. It is important to check the tunnel and paracentesis sites for the presence of vitreous. A cyclodialysis spatula can be used to sweep any vitreal strands centrally and away from the wound.

5. Pars plana support. If there is a significant amount of phacodonesis, consider stabilizing the lens posteriorly. A sclerotomy 3 to 4 mm posterior to the limbus is made, and a Koch spatula introduced to stabilize the lens from behind the posterior capsule. Be careful not to angle the spatula too far posteriorly to avoid displacing the vitreous. This maneuver should only be performed by experienced surgeons.

Immediate Postoperative Medications

In the setting of multiple ocular surgeries, consider a subconjunctival injection of antibiotics and steroids to minimize inflammation and risk of infection.

RELEVANT POSTOPERATIVE ISSUES

Complications

1. Postoperative IOP elevation. This can be caused by retained viscoelastic material, which is more common when minimal aspiration is used in order to prevent extension of zonular dehiscence. Postoperative acetazolamide and topical aqueous suppressants can be used to lower IOP. For very high IOP, consider tapping the paracentesis site. If performing this technique, avoid copious release of fluid that can suddenly shallow the anterior chamber, prolapse vitreous, or shift the IOL.

2. IOL malposition. Repositioning may be required for patients with subjective complaints or persistent intraocular inflammation.

3. Dislocated PCIOL. May require removal by a retina surgeon via a pars plana approach.

4. Retained crystalline lens fragments. Small amounts of cortical material in the posterior segment usually do not require further intervention. However, large cortical or nuclear fragments should be removed by an experienced retina surgeon within 7 to 10 days.

5. Persistent corneal edema. Consider intensive treatment with a topical steroid (prednisolone acetate 1% one to two drops every 1 to 2 hours). Consider NSAIDs (eg, ketorolac 0.5% [Acular] or diclofenac 0.1% [Voltaren]). However, use NSAIDs sparingly in the case of corneal epithelial compromise since there have been reports of corneal epithelial toxicity with these medications.

6. CME (see Appendix C).

7. Retinal detachment.

Postoperative Medications

1. Consider treatment with NSAIDs (eg, ketorolac 0.5% [Acular] or diclofenac 0.1% [Voltaren]) and topical antibiotics.

2. If a capsular rupture has occurred, refer to Appendix C for treatment options.

Follow-Up

1. Early dilated examination (within the first week) should be performed to evaluate for IOL centration, retained lens fragments, retinal complications, and CME.

2. Frequent follow-ups may be necessary for IOP measurement due to traumatic glaucoma or retained viscoelastic.

WHEN TO CONSIDER ALTERNATIVE PROCEDURES

1. Inadequately controlled glaucoma. Consider phacoemulsification combined with a glaucoma procedure.

2. Uncontrolled inflammation. Postpone surgery until inflammation is well-controlled, except in the case of phacoantigenic uveitis.

3. Phacodonesis, iridodonesis, and lens subluxation. Consider ICCE or ECCE.

4. Zonular rupture >6 clock hours (50%). Consider ICCE.

5. Posterior capsular break. Lens removal should be performed through a pars plana approach, especially if there is lens material beyond the posterior capsule in the posterior segment.

6. Previous pars plana vitrectomy. Consider ECCE.

7. Reduced ERG secondary to IOFB. Consider deferring surgery.

8. Traumatic optic neuropathy. Consider deferring surgery.

KEY POINTS

1. Defer elective cataract surgery until the eye has stabilized from the trauma and any surgical repairs.

2. *If the posterior segment cannot be clearly visualized, a B-scan is required to rule out a retinal detachment or IOFB.*

3. Preoperative presence of an RAPD or visual acuity of light perception without projection suggests advanced retinal and/or optic nerve pathology, which will probably limit useful visual recovery (reconsider need for cataract surgery).

4. Begin prophylactic anti-inflammatory treatment for CME prior to surgery (see Appendix C).

5. Measure pupillary dilation. Perform surgical dilation if pharmacologic dilation is inadequate.

6. Optimize management of IOP before surgery.

7. Avoid topical anesthesia, Honan balloon, Super-Pinky, and digital massage.

8. The use of dye to stain the anterior capsule provides excellent visibility of the leading edge of the capsulorrhexis (see Chapter 10).

9. Avoid hyperinflation of the anterior chamber.

10. Minimize displacement of the lens throughout surgery. Avoid tractional forces directed away from suspected regions of zonular weakness points.

11. Verify zonular stability prior to placing an IOL.

12. If zonular instability is suspected, perform an early dilated examination to assess IOL positioning and support if zonular instability is suspected.

REFERENCES

1. Blum M, Tetz MR, Greiner C, et al. Treatment of traumatic cataracts. *J Cataract Refract Surg.* 1996;22(3):342-346.

2. Krishnamachary M, Rathi V, Gupta S. Management of traumatic cataract in children. *J Cataract Refract Surg.* 1997;23(Suppl1):681-687.

3. Jonas JB, Knorr HL, Budde WM. Prognostic factors in ocular injuries caused by intraocular or retrobulbar foreign bodies. *Ophthalmology.* 2000;107(5):823-828.

4. Apple DJ, Federman JL, Krolicki TJ, et al. Irreversible silicone oil adhesion to silicone intraocular lenses. *Ophthalmology.* 1996;103:1555-1562.

5. Fine IH, Hoffman RS. Phacoemulsification in the presence of pseudoexfoliation: challenges and options. *J Cataract Refract Surg.* 1997;23:160-65.

6. Lee V, Bloom P. Microhook capsule stabilization for phacoemulsification in eyes with pseudoexfoliation-syndrome-induced lens stability. *J Cataract Refract Surg.* 1999;25:1567-70.

THE POSTERIOR POLAR CATARACT

Victor L. Perez, MD
Roberto Pineda II, MD

RELEVANT PREOPERATIVE ISSUES

Clinical Settings

Posterior polar cataracts are congenital lens opacities located in the central posterior cortex and subcapsular area. These cataracts typically present as dense white opacities with a characteristic concentric "whorl-like" pattern and central thickening.[1] Posterior polar cataracts can be bilateral and are commonly inherited in an autosomal dominant pattern. The locus has been mapped to the human chromosome 20p12-q12.[2] Microphthalmia, glaucoma, myopia, and other systemic abnormalities such as diabetes insipidus, diabetes mellitus, optic nerve atrophy, and deafness (DIDMOAD) can be found in patients with polar cataracts.[3,4] These cataracts have been postulated to occur because of lens invasion by mesoblastic tissue or persistence of the hyaloid artery.[5] Therefore, detailed examination of the anterior vitreous is important to determine if any vestigeal remnants are still present. Two types of polar cataracts have been described—the stationary and the progressive. Patients with the progressive type tend to develop symptoms when the peripheral processes of the concentric cataract enlarge. Alternatively, patients with the stationary type are more likely to develop symptoms as the density of the cataract increases, or age-related pupillary miosis develops.[5] These changes usually develop between the ages of 30 to 40, despite the fact that the opacity is present at birth.[6] The most common disabling symptom is glare caused by the scattering of light. Loss of visual acuity and contrast sensitivity can also occur.

The extraction of the posterior polar cataract is not a routine procedure. This cataract's intimate association with the posterior capsule and the presence of abnormal capsular thinning increase the risk of posterior capsular complications and make phacoemulsification a surgical challenge.

Risks and Complications

Patients with a posterior polar cataract may have greater incidences of the following complications:

1. Posterior capsular rupture (26% to 36%).[5,6]

2. Vitreous loss.

3. CME from capsular complications.

4. Loss of nuclear fragments into the posterior segment.

5. Posterior capsule residual plaque.

6. IOL subluxation.

Pertinent History

In addition to the usual ophthalmic history, surgeons should pay particular attention to the following:

1. Visually significant glare.

2. History of vision changes in the fellow eye.

3. History of other systemic disorders (eg, diabetes).

4. Family history of congenital cataracts.

5. History of complications during cataract surgery in the fellow eye.

Clinical Evaluation

The preoperative evaluation should include a comprehensive eye examination, with consideration of the following points, depending on the specific pathology:

1. Glare testing (eg, brightness acuity testing [BAT]).

2. Careful and detailed examination of the lens and opacity. It is very important to assess the location of the lens opacity and any association with an anterior vitreous abnormality.

3. Dilated fundoscopic examination to assess the status of the optic nerve (eg, optic atrophy or Bergmeister's papilla).

4. Consider examination of family members for posterior polar cataracts.

STRATEGIES TO MAXIMIZE OUTCOMES

1. Defer cataract surgery until the patient's visual complaints are truly troublesome.

2. To maximize patient satisfaction and promote realistic expectations, discuss any specific risks and complications of cataract surgery that are relevant to your patient. Focus on the risk of capsular rupture and its complications, including IOL placement issues.

3. Use CME prophylaxis medications (see Appendix C).

4. Be prepared to perform an anterior vitrectomy. In fact, schedule the surgery as cataract extraction with vitrectomy.

PERIOPERATIVE CONSIDERATIONS AND TECHNIQUES

Immediate Preoperative Medications

1. Maximize pupillary dilation with phenylephrine 2.5% to 10% plus tropicamide 1% every 10 minutes x 3, starting 1 hour prior to surgery.

2. Consider the use of topical steroids and NSAIDs preoperatively for CME prophylaxis (see Appendix C).

Anesthesia Considerations

A peribulbar block is an excellent choice in these cases because it minimizes positive pressure on the vitreous and forward movement of the posterior capsule. Topical anesthesia should be avoided in order to prevent unexpected ocular movements with concomitant positive vitreous pressure. For the same reason, ocular compression (with digital massage or a device such as a Honan balloon or Super-Pinky) is advocated after application of local anesthesia to promote hypotony.

Wound Construction

While a small, clear corneal incision can be safely performed, a scleral tunnel approach is recommended due to the high risk of capsular complications and the possible need for conversion to extracapsular extraction.

Pupillary Considerations

A well-dilated pupil is important in order to optimize visualization of the polar cataract and to evaluate its behavior when the capsule is manipulated.

Capsulorrhexis and Other Capsular Considerations

An anterior capsulorrhexis often can be performed using a standard technique. The size of the capsulorrhexis is important. It should be small enough to ensure enough anterior capsular support for a sulcus-fixated IOL if necessary. However, if the capsulorrhexis is too small it may increase hydrostatic pressure on the bag during hydrodelineation, predisposing to capsular rupture.

Hydrodissection

Hydrodissection is contraindicated in these patients. The area where the polar cataract is adhered to the posterior capsule represents a point of weakness. If hydrodissection is performed, the fluid wave will cause a hydraulic rupture of the posterior capsule at this point, and a tear can then extend peripherally.[6]

Hydrodelineation

Cortical cleaving with hydrodissection is contraindicated. However, hydrodelineation is mandatory.[6] With this technique, an epinuclear bowl will be created, providing protection to the capsule during phacoemulsification. Gentle, minimal nuclear rotation, or no nuclear rotation, is encouraged in order to minimize tractional forces between the polar cataract and the posterior capsule (Figure 12-1).

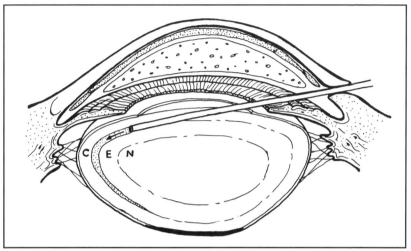

Figure 12-1. Hydrodelineation should be performed in the posterior polar cataract. Hydrodissection is contraindicated. Additionally, posterior capsular polishing is not recommended due to an abnormally thin posterior capsule and high rate of capsular rupture.

Phacoemulsification

Maintaining the AC Depth

- It is very important to minimize stress on the capsule during phacoemulsifica-tion. Fluctuations in the AC depth should be minimized in order to prevent forward movement of the capsule and vitreous:
  - Generous use of viscoelastic material will keep the anterior chamber well formed, especially during the introduction and removal of instruments from the eye.
  - Minimize repetitive removal and re-introduction of instruments, as this may cause the anterior chamber to collapse.
  - Some surgeons advocate placement of additional viscoelastic in the anteri-or chamber each time instruments are removed from the eye to prevent for-ward displacement of the anterior capsule and vitreous.
  - The infusion bottle should be kept at a low height to prevent overdisten-sion of the posterior capsule.

Removal of Nucleus

We generally prefer a chopping technique over nuclear fractis (divide-and-con-quer technique) because there is less stress on the posterior capsule. However, since many of these patients are younger, chopping may be difficult due to the softness of the nucleus. In this case, it may be necessary to bowl out the central nucleus using low aspiration and vacuum, taking care to leave the epinuclear layer intact.

Cortical (Epinuclear) Aspiration

Epinuclear Removal

- Special attention should be paid to removal of the epinucleus. It is critical to begin removing the epinucleus from the peripheral cortex, with minimal traction on the central plate. Stripping should be performed 360 degrees at the periphery, with the central zone left attached until the last stage of the aspiration.[6] We recommend splitting the irrigation and aspiration ports to perform bimanual irrigation and aspiration. A manual irrigation and aspiration device is an excellent alternative.

Central Adhesions

Be prepared to encounter two possible scenarios:

- Central plaque or haze. Do not perform capsular polishing or capsular vacuuming ("cap-vac"), and do not attempt to remove the plaque. This can be removed during Nd:YAG at a later date. Proceed with placement of the IOL.

- Posterior capsular rupture. This can present as a circular hole, a radial tear, or a combination of both. It is important to minimize changes in the depth of the anterior chamber that would cause the vitreous to move forward through the rupture. Do not remove the aspiration instrument from the eye without first stabilizing the vitreous. This can be done by injecting viscoelastic at the rupture site with your second hand through the paracentesis incision and pushing the vitreous posteriorly. Then remove the aspiration instrument carefully to prevent vitreous prolapse. It is sometimes possible to convert a posterior tear into a CCC. When possible, this is desirable since a posterior CCC is more stable and may permit endocapsular IOL placement.

Special Techniques

Anterior Vitrectomy

- We suggest two-port vitrectomy to manage capsular ruptures with vitreous prolapse into the anterior chamber. The infusion cannula can be used separately and directed away from the capsular defect into the peripheral anterior angle. This will lessen turbulence at the cutter tip and reduce hydration of the vitreous, thereby lowering the risk of capsular tear extension. The vitrector should be used with a high cutting rate and low vacuum/aspiration flow rates (eg, cut rate = 400 cuts/min, vacuum = 100 mmHg, aspiration = 5 cc/min). Vitrectomy should be carried out with slow and circumferential movements, beginning with the anterior chamber and moving toward the capsular bag and close to the area of the rupture. Distortion of the pupillary margin should alert the surgeon to persistent vitreous material in the anterior chamber. It is important to check the tunnel and paracentesis sites for the presence of vitreous. A cyclodialysis spatula can be used to sweep any vitreal strands centrally, away from the wound.

IOL Implantation

1. If there is no posterior capsular rupture, the IOL can be placed safely in the capsular bag.

2. If there is a posterior capsular rupture, an IOL sometimes can be placed in the sulcus, depending upon how much capsular support is present. Some surgeons recommend anchoring a sulcus-fixated lens by prolapsing the optic behind the anterior capsulorrhexis while the haptics remain in the sulcus.

3. When placing foldable IOLs (with or without posterior capsular rupture), acrylic IOLs are a good choice since they allow slow unfolding with less stress to the capsule, giving the surgeon greater control. Crease the lens implant on the long axis so that the trailing haptic remains outside the wound after unfolding. Unfold the lens in the anterior chamber very slowly, then slide the leading haptic into place.

4. If there is insufficient support for a sulcus-fixated lens, consider a sutured posterior chamber IOL or anterior chamber IOL, depending on the surgeon's experience.

5. After IOL implantation, a manual irrigation and aspiration (eg, Simcoe) or vitrector can be used for gentle, controlled removal of residual viscoelastic with less stress on the capsule.

RELEVANT POSTOPERATIVE ISSUES

Complications

1. Postoperative IOP elevation. This can be caused by retained viscoelastic material, which is more common when minimal aspiration is used in order to prevent extension of the capsular tear. Postoperative acetazolamide and topical aqueous suppressants can be used to lower the pressure. For very high IOP, consider tapping the paracentesis site. If performing this maneuver, avoid copious release of fluid that can suddenly shallow the AC, prolapse the vitreous, or shift the IOL.

2. Inflammation from residual cortical material.

3. Posterior capsular residual plaque. Consider Nd:YAG. This procedure should not be considered before 3 months postoperatively, due to the risk of retinal detachment.

4. IOL malposition. Reposition may be required for patients with subjective complaints or persistent intraocular inflammation.

5. Retained crytalline lens fragments. Small amounts of cortical material in the posterior segment usually do not require further intervention. However, large cortical or nuclear fragments should be removed by an experienced retina surgeon.

6. CME (see Appendix C).

Postoperative Medications

1. Consider treatment with a topical steroid, NSAIDs (eg, ketorolac 0.5% [Acular] or diclofenac 0.1% [Voltaren]) and topical antibiotics.
2. If capsular rupture has occurred, refer to Appendix C for treatment options.

Follow-Up

1. Frequent follow-ups may be necessary for IOP.
2. Early dilated examination (within the first week) should be performed to evaluate for IOL centration, retained lens fragments, posterior capsular opacity (PCO), and CME.

WHEN TO CONSIDER ALTERNATIVE PROCEDURES

1. Posterior polar cataract with an extensive anterior vitreal involvement. Consider pars plana lensectomy and vitrectomy with sutured PCIOL.
2. Amblyopia. Avoid surgery unless significant functional improvement can be anticipated.

KEY POINTS

1. Defer cataract surgery until the patient's visual symptoms are very troublesome.
2. Posterior capsular rupture is a common complication (26% to 36%).
3. Avoid hydrodissection.
4. Use hydrodelineation.
5. Use all available techniques to minimize stress on the capsule.
6. Keep the infusion bottle height low.
7. Maintain a stable anterior chamber.
8. Strip epinuclear material from the periphery first and remove the central area last.
9. Be prepared for an anterior vitrectomy.

REFERENCES

1. Eshagian J. Human posterior subcapsular cataracts. *Trans Ophthal Soc UK*. 1982;102:364-368.
2. Yamada K, Yoshiura K, Kondo S, et al. An autosomal dominant posterior polar cataract locus maps to human chromosome 20p12-q12. *Eur J Hum Genet*. 2000;8(7):535-539.
3. Greeves RA. Two cases of microphthalmia. *Trans Ophthalmol Soc UK*. 1914;34:289-300.
4. Bekir NA, Gungor K, Guran S. A DIDMOAD syndrome family with juvenile glaucoma and myopia findings. *Acta Ophthalmol Scand*. 2000;78(4):480-482.
5. Osher RH, Koch DD. Posterior polar cataracts: a predisposition to intraoperative posterior capsular rupture. *J Cataract Refract Surg*. 1990;16:157-162.
6. Vasavada A. Phacoemulsification in eyes with posterior polar cataract. *J Cataract Refract Surg*. 1999;25:238-244.

13

THE DIABETIC PATIENT

Sabera Shah, MD
Alejandro Espaillat, MD
Lloyd M. Aiello, MD

RELEVANT PREOPERATIVE ISSUES

Clinical Setting

Diabetes is becoming more common. It is estimated that its global prevalence will double from 110 million to 221 million between 1994 and 2010.[1] Cataracts are more prevalent in patients with diabetes. There is a three- to four-fold excess prevalence in patients younger than 65 years old, and up to two-fold excess prevalence in those above 64 years old.[2] Cataract is an important cause of visual loss in diabetes. In the Wisconsin epidemiological study of diabetic retinopathy (WESDR), cataract was the most common cause of legal blindness in older-onset diabetics, and the second most common cause in younger-onset diabetics.[3]

The incidence of cataract surgery is higher in patients with diabetes. The 10-year cumulative incidence of cataract surgery in patients with diabetes in the WESDR was two to five times higher than in a comparable nondiabetic population.[4] Visual acuity after cataract surgery in diabetes may be poor[5,6] and the incidence of complications high.[7] Indications for cataract surgery in diabetic patients include the need for visual rehabilitation and the need for visualization of the posterior segment for evaluation and treatment.

Risks and Complications

Diabetic patients may have greater incidences of the following complications:

1. Intraoperative and postoperative hyphema from rubeosis and increased vascular fragility.
2. Intraoperative and postoperative corneal edema.
3. Postoperative corneal epitheliopathy.
4. Postoperative inflammation.
5. Increased IOP.
6. Iris trauma, capsular tear, and vitreous loss (from a small pupil).

7. Progression of diabetic retinopathy.

8. Clinically significant macular edema (CSME).

9. Epiretinal membrane formation.

10. Sterile endophthalmitis.

Pertinent History

In addition to the usual ophthalmic history, surgeons should pay particular attention to the following:

1. Control of systemic diabetes.

2. Visual function of the fellow eye.

3. Level of diabetic retinopathy.

4. History of neovascular glaucoma.

5. History of vitrectomy/retinal surgery.

6. History of CSME or proliferative diabetic retinopathy (PDR).

7. History of recurrent erosions or corneal disease.

8. Ocular and systemic medications (especially miotics).

9. Outcome of cataract surgery in the other eye.

10. Determine if the patient has any risk factors for progression of diabetic retinopathy after cataract extraction:
    - Duration and type of diabetes mellitus (DM)
    - Glycemic control levels of HbA1c
    - Cholesterol level
    - Coronary artery disease
    - Blood pressure
    - Renal disease
    - Anemia

Clinical Evaluation

The preoperative evaluation should include a comprehensive eye examination, with consideration of the following points, depending on the specific pathology:

1. Visual function evaluation:
   - Determine potential visual acuity using the potential acuity meter (PAM), pinhole acuity potential (PAP), or laser interferometry to estimate visual outcome
   - Optional contrast sensitivity testing should be considered

2. Anterior segment examination:
   - Evaluate integrity of the corneal epithelium
   - Evaluate the pupil size, as well as any neovascularization of the iris

- Evaluate the angle structures with gonioscopy
- Determine the type and degree of the cataract

3. Dilated fundoscopic examination:
   - Establish the level of diabetic retinopathy and determine the presence of CSME

STRATEGIES TO MAXIMIZE OUTCOMES

1. To maximize patient satisfaction and promote realistic expectations, discuss any specific risks and complications of cataract surgery listed in the Risks and Complications section that are relevant to your patient. Also discuss reasonable expectations for visual outcome and other benefits of surgery, the need for pre- and postoperative laser treatment, postoperative course and healing time, and choice of IOL implant.

2. Discuss potential risk factors with the patient's other health care providers. Control the patient's systemic disease as well as possible.

3. Treat active retinopathy and macular edema when possible and indicated before the cataract extraction. Considerations for laser treatment include:
   - PDR with high-risk characteristics
   - PDR without high-risk characteristics but with significant nonperfusion
   - Moderate to severe nonproliferative diabetic retinopathy (NPDR) with significant nonperfusion, along with high-risk systemic factors (control of blood sugar, hypertension, anemia, and renal disease) for progression of retinopathy after the cataract surgery

4. For early macular edema and CSME, use fluorescein angiography to determine treatable lesions and focal laser surgery if indicated. Postpone cataract surgery if possible and re-evaluate the macula in 3 to 4 months. Reconsider cataract surgery when the macular edema has resolved.

5. Lens choices should include an IOL with a 6.0 mm optic or larger to allow a better visualization of the retina for future laser treatment.

PERIOPERATIVE CONSIDERATIONS AND TECHNIQUES

Immediate Preoperative Medications

Maximize preoperative pupillary dilation (phenylephrine 2.5% to 10%, tropicamide 1% or cyclopentolate 0.5% to 1%, and flurbiprofen 0.03% or ketorolac tromethamine 0.5% every 10 minutes x 3, starting 1 hour prior to surgery).

It is generally recommended that patients do not take oral hypoglycemic medications on the day of surgery, and that they take half of their NPH (neutral protein Hagedon) insulin and no regular insulin on the day of surgery. Alternatively, management of the patient's blood sugar can be guided by the preoperative and postoperative glucose levels.

Anesthesia Considerations

Because maintaining glucose levels is challenging in fasting diabetics, we recommend scheduling cataract surgery early in the morning for diabetic patients. If extensive pupil manipulation is anticipated (ie, for miotic pupils), avoid topical/intracameral anesthesia.

Wound Construction

Consider a scleral tunnel/limbal approach. Patients affected with diabetes mellitus may already have compromised corneas. These corneas may not tolerate a clear corneal incision well, leading to delayed healing, corneal edema, wound leak, and possible infection. A scleral tunnel incision is especially necessary in patients who may require panretinal photocoagulation in the immediate postoperative period. This is due to the need for a clear view through the cornea, as well as to the possibility of endophthalmitis or corneal epithelial trauma when placing a contact lens on a fresh clear corneal incision. It is advantageous to select the temporal quadrant for scleral tunnel incision, leaving the superior quadrant intact for possible future filtration procedures or shunts should the patient develop neovascular glaucoma.

Viscoelastic Considerations

Use high molecular weight cohesive viscoelastic (Amvisc Plus, Healon, or Healon GV) to maximize pupillary dilation and to aid in hemostasis.

Pupillary Considerations

Patients with longstanding diabetes may develop an ischemic, spastic pupil with secondary poor dilation. A fibrotic ring may develop around the pupil due to regressed rubeosis. The pupil should be dilated mechanically and with liberal use of viscoelastics. Avoid excessive manipulation of the iris to prevent hyphema and postoperative inflammation. If the pupil is less than 6.0 mm, see Chapter 3.

Glycogen deposits in the pigment epithelium cause release of pigments with the slightest manipulation. With this phenomenon, the iris becomes floppy and loose, thus increasing the risk of damaging the iris with either a phaco tip or with an irrigation and aspiration cannula. To prevent damaging the iris, inject a bead of viscoelastic at the wound site prior to re-entering the eye each time.

Capsulorrhexis and Other Capsular Considerations

A large capsulorrhexis is recommended to accommodate a large-optic IOL. In the presence of anterior capsular rim opacification, a large capsulorrhexis will enable better visualization of the retina and facilitate peripheral laser treatment.

Hydrodissection

1. Patients who previously had vitreoretinal surgery may have very weak zonules. To avoid any stress to the zonules, a careful hydrodissection is crucial. Sometimes it is safer to prolapse the nucleus in the anterior chamber and complete the phacoemulsification at the iris plane.

2. One technique to perform hydrodissection is to use a 26-gauge blunt cannula to elevate the anterior capsular flap away from the cortical material. The can-

nula will maintain the anterior capsule in a tented-up position at the injection site. To ensure an effective fluid wave, it is important to insert the cannula far enough toward the equator to prevent reflux of fluid along the cannula barrel. Once the cannula is properly placed and the anterior capsule is elevated, continuous, gentle irrigation will create the fluid wave and cleave the cortex from the posterior capsule in most locations. Repeating the hydrodissection in multiple quadrants is helpful. Make sure that the lens can spin freely within the capsular bag before proceeding with phacoemulsification.

3. If excessive lens mobility is noted on hydrodissection, it is advisable to convert to ECCE to prevent the nucleus or lens fragments from dropping into the vitreous, vitreous loss, and other serious complications that may require additional surgery at a later date.

Phacoemulsification

Any of the standard phacoemulsification techniques can be used to remove the cataract; however, to minimize phaco energy transmitted to the corneal endothelium, a chopping technique may be preferred over a nuclear fractis (divide-and-conquer) technique depending upon lens density and capsular integrity. Phacoemulsification at the pupillary plane or "in-the-bag" will avoid damage to the corneal endothelium.

Cortical Aspiration

Thorough cortical clean-up should be performed after phacoemulsification because of the high incidence of posterior capsular opacity in patients with diabetes. A Kuglen hook or similar instrument can be used to retract the pupil, allowing direct visualization of any remaining cortical material. Careful polishing of the posterior capsule and under the surface of the anterior capsule rim may also prevent PCO (see Figure 5-2).

IOL Implantation

A foldable acrylic or PMMA IOL with at least a 6.0-mm optic or larger is preferable for diabetic eyes. Silicone IOLs are not a good choice if the patient is likely to undergo an air/fluid exchange (due to condensation)[8] or require a vitreous substitute such as silicone oil (due to irreversible silicone oil adhesion to the silicone IOL).[9] Furthermore, the literature has indicated that silicone IOLs may stimulate inflammation in diabetic eyes.

Special Techniques

Intraocular Diathermy for Iris Neovascularization

In the past, diathermy had been applied sparingly to the pupillary margin 360 degrees to minimize bleeding from neovascular vessels on the iris and to release pupillary membranes. Additional coagulation of large vessels was also performed. This procedure allowed pupillary manipulation without excessive intraocular hemorrhage. However, this technique is rarely employed today and can be avoided by proper management of iris neovascularization before cataract surgery.

RELEVANT POSTOPERATIVE ISSUES

Complications

1. Ocular infection. Fortunately, these complications are infrequent. Diabetic eyes with poor circulation have a tendency to develop sterile endophthalmitis. Any symptoms such as ocular pain, increased redness, change in vision, excessive inflammation in the anterior chamber and/or vitreous clouding should be taken seriously. Prompt consultation with a retinal specialist is warranted.

2. Hyphema. Manipulation of the iris or pupil in the presence of active rubeosis or angle neovascularization could cause hyphema during the postoperative period. Although the hyphema usually resolves spontaneously, attention should be paid to possible sequelae, such as increased IOP and intraocular inflammation.

3. Inflammation. Diabetic eyes are prone to develop excessive postoperative inflammation. The prolonged use of topical steroids can help prevent serious problems.

4. Increased IOP. A minimal IOP spike for the first 2 days after cataract surgery is common. Diabetic eyes with compromised circulation do not tolerate pressure of 25 to 30 mmHg even for a few days and require treatment.

5. PCO. The incidence of PCO is slightly higher in patients with diabetes. The presentation of PCO may be delayed by careful polishing of the posterior capsule and rim of the anterior capsule, as well as by meticulous removal of the cortex during aspiration. This will allow a clearer view of the retina for evaluation and/or laser treatment, if needed. Nd:YAG laser capsulotomy should be avoided until absolutely necessary due to the increased risk of CME in diabetics.

6. Diabetic retinopathy. A poor visual outcome after successful and uneventful cataract surgery is most commonly related to the retinal complications of diabetic retinopathy. Careful evaluation of the level of retinopathy and laser treatment prior to cataract surgery may achieve the maximum possible outcome. If there is preoperative evidence of active PDR or severe NPDR, immediate dilated fundus examination is required (within a 1 week period) to determine the need for additional panretinal photocoagulation (see Appendix D).

7. CME. The presence of macular edema poses a challenge during the first 3 months of the postoperative period. Severe nonperfusion, waxy exudates, and multiple microaneurysms may suggest diabetic macular edema. However, sometimes it is impossible to differentiate between diabetic macular edema and CME. In this case, if there is no significant deterioration of visual acuity in the immediate postoperative period, it is advisable to postpone treatment. The persistence of macular edema after 3 months requires fluorescein angiography and focal laser treatment if CSME is diagnosed (see Appendix C).

Postoperative Medications

Consider routine treatment with a topical steroid, NSAIDs (eg, ketorolac 0.5% [Acular] or diclofenac 0.1% [Voltaren]), and topical antibiotics.

Follow-Up

1. Patients with surgical complications, and those with active retinopathy may require multiple follow-up visits. During the first postoperative day, resume any systemic medications. Special attention should be paid to IOP the first week after surgery.

2. Dilated fundoscopy is often recommended 1 week, 3 to 4 weeks, 6 weeks, and 3 months after cataract surgery, to assess the progression of diabetic retinopathy and the need for laser treatment.

WHEN TO CONSIDER ALTERNATIVE PROCEDURES

1. In cases of high-risk PDR with vitreous hemorrhage and cataracts, consider a pars plana lensectomy, vitrectomy, endolaser, and an IOL implant.

2. In cases of neovascular glaucoma with high IOPs and cataracts, panretinal photocoagulation and cryoablation is recommended prior to cataract surgery. Also, consider a glaucoma shunt procedure at the time of the cataract surgery.

3. If pupil dilation yields inadequate visualization, consider converting to an extracapsular cataract extraction technique. Consider conversion particularly in cases of dense nuclear sclerosis and pseudoexfoliation in which there is an increased risk of capsular disruption.

KEY POINTS

1. Control of systemic diabetes is critical.

2. High-risk PDR and CSME should be treated before cataract surgery.

3. Obtain maximal pharmacologic dilation prior to surgery.

4. Have a low threshold to enlarge the pupil.

5. Consider an acrylic or PMMA IOL instead of a silicone IOL.

6. Dilated fundus examination should be performed postoperatively as soon as possible to determine the level of retinopathy.

7. Postoperative photocoagulation should be performed as soon as possible, when indicated.

8. Be sure to discuss with the patient what are reasonable expectations for visual outcome in the context of his or her level of diabetic retinopathy.

REFERENCES

1. Amos AF, McCarty DJ, Zimmet P. The rising global burden of diabetes and its complications: estimates and projections to the year 2010. *Diab Med.* 1997;14:81-85.
2. Ederer F, Hiller R. Senile lens changes and diabetes in two population studies. *Am J Ophthalmol.* 1981;91:381-95.
3. Klein R, Klein BE, Moss SE. Visual impairment in diabetes. *Ophthalmology.* 1984;91:1-9.
4. Klein BE, Klein R, Moss SE. Incidence of cataract surgery in the Wisconsin epidemiologic study of diabetic retinopathy. *Am J Ophthalmol.* 1995;119:295-300.

5. Schatz H, Atienza D, McDonald HR, et al. Severe diabetic retinopathy after cataract surgery. *Am J Ophthalmol*. 1994;117:314-21.

6. Pollack A, Leiba H, Bukelman A, et al. The course of diabetic retinopathy following cataract surgery in eyes previously treated with laser photocoagulation. *Br J Ophthalmol*. 1992;76:228-31.

7. Krupsky S, Zalish M, Oliver M, Pollack A. Anterior segment complications in diabetic patients following extracapsular cataract extraction and posterior chamber intraocular lens implantation. *Ophthalmic Surg*. 1991;22:526-30.

8. Hainsworth DP, Chen SN, Cox TA, Jaffe GJ. Condensation on polymethylmethacrylate, acrylic polymer, and silicone intraocular lenses after fluid-air exchange in rabbits. *Ophthalmology*. 1996;103:1410-1418.

9. Apple DJ, Federman JL, Krolicki TJ, et al. Irreversible silicone oil adhesion to silicone intraocular lenses. *Ophthalmology*. 1996;103:1555-1562.

14

THE PEDIATRIC CATARACT

Kailenn Tsao, MD
Melanie Kazlas, MD

RELEVANT PREOPERATIVE ISSUES

Clinical Settings

The prevalence of visually significant pediatric cataracts is estimated to be as high as 5.6/10,000. As many as 40,000 children are blind from cataracts worldwide.[1] One-third of bilateral cataracts in the pediatric population are inherited, one-third are idiopathic, and one-third are related to a systemic abnormality.[2]

Cataracts in the pediatric population challenge the surgeon with respect to diagnosis, preoperative preparation, surgical technique, and postoperative management. Additional ocular abnormalities are common; the surgeon should be prepared to encounter amblyopia (50%), glaucoma (30%), strabismus (>50%), and secondary membranes (100%).[3] Systemic abnormalities should be suspected in bilateral cataracts and are appropriately managed in conjunction with a pediatric specialist. Unilateral cataracts in an otherwise healthy child require no further work-up.

Cataracts in the preverbal population require special assessment of severity of the opacity, since surgery may be delayed or avoided in milder cases. The morphology of the cataract can indicate the prognosis for vision. For example, an anterior polar cataract is commonly unilateral, less than 2 mm, and nonprogressive with excellent prognosis without surgery.[4] Partial or lamellar cataracts may have less of an effect on the developing visual system and may be treated with pupillary dilation.

If the cataract is visually significant, it is critical to proceed with surgery as soon as possible, ideally within the first 2 months of life, in order to lessen the risk of amblyopia.[5] Visually significant cataracts include those that occupy 3 mm or more of the embryonal and fetal nucleus, and those that obscure the view of retinal vessels with the direct ophthalmoscope through an undilated pupil. Extraction of visually significant bilateral cataracts should commence within 1 week of diagnosis and should not be separated by more than 1 week in time. Unilateral or asymmetric cataracts require expeditious extraction within 1 week of diagnosis to minimize amblyopia.

IOL implantation in children has been the subject of intense interest over the last decade. Although the FDA has not approved IOLs in children under 18, many surgeons now implant IOLs in children as young as 2 years of age, thereby greatly simplifying amblyopia management. New IOLs have been designed with children in mind and are available in Europe. Creative solutions have been proposed to lessen problems related to myopic shift during childhood, PCO, and capsular contraction. More studies are needed to evaluate the risks and benefits of pediatric IOL use, especially in young children.

Risks and Complications

Pediatric patients may have greater incidences of several complications:

1. General anesthesia is usually necessary in the pediatric population. The systemic health of the child or infant should be weighed against the risks of the anesthesia, which may be exaggerated if the child has other systemic abnormalities.

2. Even with successful surgery, visual outcomes may often be poor because of complications of amblyopia. Strict compliance with eye patching is critical.

3. Complications related to IOLs are increased in children and include uveitis, glaucoma, capsular opacification, and IOL power miscalculations. Secondary surgery may be required, or a secondary implant may be placed if the child is left aphakic.

4. Myopic shifts may require a second surgery (eg, IOL exchange, piggyback lens placement) or other refractive treatment (eg, glasses, contact lenses).

5. Complications related to systemic or other ocular abnormalities may limit potential vision and may obviate the benefit of surgery.

Pertinent History

In addition to the usual ophthalmic history, surgeons should pay particular attention to the following:

1. Check parents and siblings for evidence of cataracts.

2. Inquire about previous history of cataractogenic steroid use.

3. Pregnancy, birth history, and medical history may provide clues to cataract etiology. Poorly or inadequately treated diabetes may cause pediatric cataract with life-threatening complications. Inquire about intrauterine infection.

4. Ocular trauma is a major cause of unilateral cataract.

5. Family history of malignant hyperthermia or homocystinuria may be associated with life-threatening intraoperative complications.[2]

Clinical Evaluation

The preoperative evaluation should include a comprehensive eye examination, with consideration of the following points, depending on the specific pathology:

1. Baseline laboratory studies include electrolytes, urine reducing substances and amino acids, chromosomal studies, screening antibody panel titers for infection, audiograms, iron and calcium levels, and galactokinase.[4]

2. Clinical examination of the preverbal child is difficult, but the host of possible associated ocular abnormalities mandates careful attention to all components of the ophthalmic exam. A low threshold for examination under anesthesia is necessary to avoid missing serious treatable entities.

3. Visual acuity and careful refraction.

4. External exam. Characteristic faces and physical deformities may be seen in chromosomal trisomies, Hallermann-Streiff syndrome, Alport's syndrome, metabolic storage diseases, neurofibromatosis type 2, and Marfan's syndrome.[4]

5. Anterior segment dimensions. Routine ocular measurements of corneal diameter and axial length may detect microcornea, microphthalmos, staphylomas, and persistent hyperplastic primary vitreous (PHPV). Axial length and keratometry measurements will be required if an IOL is contemplated.

6. Anterior segment. Associated anterior segment abnormalities may include corneal opacities, angle and iris abnormalities, and lens subluxation. These findings should prompt further investigation with respect to metabolic storage diseases, anterior segment dysgeneses, and Marfan's syndrome. Posterior synechiae and uveitis point toward inflammatory conditions such as infection, juvenile rheumatoid arthritis, or trauma.[2]

7. Pupillary dilation. Take note of maximal pharmacologic pupillary dilation to determine the need for pupil expanding procedures.

8. Glaucoma assessment. IOP and gonioscopic evaluation may reveal evidence of glaucoma that is associated with anterior segment dysgeneses, aniridia, spherophakia, PHPV, Stickler's syndrome, and rubella.[6]

9. Posterior segment. Posterior segment abnormalities that may be seen include PHPV, retinopathy of prematurity (ROP), vascular abnormalities (Fabry's disease), and pigmentary retinopathy (Alport's syndrome, retinitis pigmentosa, rubella, and Stickler's syndrome).[5]

10. Preoperative visual-evoked potentials (VEP) and ERG may be useful in predicting postoperative visual prognosis.

IOL Choice Considerations

1. Age of patient. Pediatric IOL implantation is rapidly gaining acceptance. Early IOL implantation has been reported to be successful and has been advocated to reduce the risk of amblyopia and aphakic glaucoma.[3,6-11] However, IOLs are usually not recommended for children under age 2, due to the rapid growth of the eye during this time. In addition, at this writing IOLs are not FDA-approved for patients younger than age 18. The Infant Aphakia Treatment Study is currently evaluating the status of IOLs in very young children.[10]

2. Lens power. Determining postoperative refractive goals remains a complex issue. There is mounting evidence to suggest that pseudophakic children undergo myopic shifts over time.[12-18] Increasingly, surgeons are aiming for residual hyperopia in young patients in order to offset these myopic shifts. Dahan and

Drusedau recommend undercorrecting by 10% in children over the age of 2 and undercorrecting by 20% in younger children.[19]

Other surgeons choose to aim for emmetropia and plan to correct future myopia with glasses, contact lenses, or laser in-situ keratomileusis (LASIK). With severe myopic shift, lens exchange may be performed. Consideration of the contralateral phakic eye also influences choice of less power.[20]

3. Materials. Acrylic lenses are the pediatric IOLs of choice for many surgeons in the United States.[6] Some studies suggest that these IOLs inhibit posterior capsule epithelial migration more than other lenses, although the data are conflicting. Acrylic IOLs have the advantage of permitting small-incision surgery. Hydrophilic acrylics such as hydroxyethylmethacrylate (HEMA) and its relatives may be the most biocompatible. Since these lenses seem to minimize adherence to intraocular tissues, they are thought to be a good choice if future explantation and IOL exchange is anticipated.

Some surgeons still prefer PMMA lenses, which have the most extensive track record for long-term safety in the human eye. Heparin-coated IOLs show promise for better compatibility in pediatric eyes but are currently available only in Europe.[9] Thinner IOL optics are useful if piggyback IOLs are contemplated; PMMA and acrylic have both been used for this purpose.

4. Size. Pediatric IOLs should be no larger than 12 mm in total diameter since even the adult ciliary sulcus only measures about 11.5 mm. IOL sizing depends on the age of the child, the corneal diameter, and whether the lens is implanted in the bag or in the sulcus.

Specially designed pediatric IOLs are not approved by the FDA but are becoming available in Europe and elsewhere. The Pullmans (Corneal, Paris, France) is a HEMA acrylic IOL with an overall diameter of 10.75 mm, suitable for children. This lens has flanges that are designed to absorb the forces of capsular bag contraction without vaulting the optic. The Coldness (IOLTECHnologie, LaRochelle, France) is specially designed for pediatric implantation. The Kidlens has an optic diameter of 5.5 mm and an overall diameter of 10.75 mm; however, the overall diameter can be compressed to fit smaller eyes. To reduce the diameter of the Kidlens IOL, the haptics are harnessed with 10-0 nylon through small eyelets and drawn closer to the optic to obtain the desired diameter. The nylon suture is then secured through eyelets in the optic.

5. Location. Primary posterior chamber IOLs have been placed in the bag and in the sulcus with good success. Secondary posterior chamber IOLs may be placed in the sulcus if the residual capsular leaflets offer sufficient support for the IOL. Some dissection may be necessary to recreate the sulcus in these cases. Sutured posterior chamber IOLs have been used if capsular support is inadequate, but the long-term safety of these lenses is uncertain.

Piggyback IOLs are emerging as a possible choice in pediatric patients, although there is little research to date to support their safety in this population. One lens is placed in the bag, while the second lens is placed anterior to the first, in the bag, or in the sulcus. As the eye matures and becomes more myopic, the second lens may be explanted.

ACIOLs are avoided at all costs because of intense postoperative inflammatory reaction, risk of angle fibrosis and glaucoma, corneal decompensation, and the changing dimensions of the angle in the growing child.[8] Secondary PCIOLs should be sutured in place.

6. Contraindications to IOL placement:
   - Children under 2 years of age (depends on surgeon)
   - Microphthalmia or microcornea
   - Aniridia
   - Glaucoma
   - Uveitis

7. Power calculations. One study has compared multiple formulas for long (>24 mm), average (22 to 24 mm), and short (<22 mm) eyes and failed to detect a difference in accuracy of predicting outcomes.[21] The four formulas compared were SRK-II, SRK-T, Holladay, and Hoffer-Q.

STRATEGIES TO MAXIMIZE OUTCOMES

1. Inform the family that a general anesthetic will be used.

2. Review with parents the absolute necessity for compliance with postoperative follow-up, therapy, and eye patching. Discuss the modalities necessary for aphakic rehabilitation, including spectacles, contact lenses, or secondary IOL placement.[7] Provide handouts explaining the procedure in lay terms to enhance compliance.

3. Prepare parents for 25 or more postoperative visits in the first year to monitor amblyopia.

4. In cases in which poor visual outcome is anticipated, prepare the family in advance, explaining reasons why the child has a low potential for vision, what steps would maximize visual rehabilitation, and the risks/benefits of surgery.

5. If IOL placement is planned, an institutional review board application and special consent form may be required by your hospital.

6. In cases of lens subluxation or lens reflux into the posterior segment, pars plana lensectomy with vitrectomy is the procedure of choice. Posterior segment complications such as PHPV or ROP may require pars plana or open sky techniques. Primary ICCE is contraindicated in the pediatric population.

7. Anticholinesterase (echothiophate) eye drops should be stopped 6 weeks prior to surgery to prevent prolonged anesthesia time.[4]

8. If the posterior segment cannot be visualized, a preoperative B-scan must be performed to rule out posterior segment pathology, including retinoblastoma.

PERIOPERATIVE CONSIDERATIONS AND TECHNIQUES

Immediate Preoperative Medications

1. Preoperative eye drops include cyclopentolate 1% (0.5% in children younger than 6 months), tropicamide 1%, and phenylephrine 2.5% administered every 5 minutes x 3, 1 hour prior to surgery to achieve maximal pupillary dilation.

2. In the absence of external blepharitis and infection, one drop of topical antibiotic such as Polytrim (Allergan, Irvine, Calif) is sufficient. In addition to the surgical preparation, place a drop of povidone iodine 5% ophthalmic solution into the inferior cul-de-sac.

3. In cases of uveitis and diabetes, consider preoperative anti-inflammatory agents, such as prednisolone acetate, and topical nonsteroidal medication.[6]

4. If a lengthy or very difficult surgery is anticipated, consider giving IV mannitol 200 mg/kg immediately prior to surgery to shrink the vitreous.

Anesthesia Considerations

Most surgeons agree that pediatric cataract surgery requires general anesthesia. Paralysis and deep anesthesia are necessary to prevent extraocular muscle contraction with traction on the less rigid sclera. Contraindications to general anesthesia are rare but may be associated with life-threatening conditions and may necessitate delaying ocular surgery even in the amblyogenic age group.

Wound Construction

Pediatric sclera is significantly less rigid than in the adult. Careful attention to anterior chamber stability is necessary to avoid anterior chamber and globe collapse. Wound construction can be carried out using a standard triplanar approach similar to the adult eye. Pars plana scleral tunneling aids in maintaining anterior chamber stability; however, a posterior limbal incision with a short tunnel facilitates maneuvering of instruments and decreases the risk of ciliary body damage and hemorrhage.

Avoid a bridle suture if possible. The suture may cause traction on the soft sclera and may mask extraocular contractions if the anesthesia becomes too light.

Viscoelastics

A cohesive viscoelastic is preferable to a dispersive viscoelastic to facilitate easy removal and prevention of postoperative IOP spikes.

Pupillary Considerations

Irides that are unresponsive to dilation drops may require lysis of the posterior synechiae, iris stretching, pupillotomy, or iris hooks (see Chapter 3).

Capsulotomy

1. The anterior capsule is highly elastic in the pediatric patient and poses challenges in the creation of the capsulotomy. Multiple capsulotomy techniques are available, each with benefits and drawbacks:

   • CCC remains the gold standard in all age groups.[22] However, achieving a large capsulorrhexis may be difficult in young patients, and radial tears are very common due to the centripetal counterforces inherent in the highly elastic capsule. Utrata forceps and a cohesive viscoelastic are recommended for precise control of the capsular leaflet. If a radial tear occurs, conversion to one of the other methods described below is highly recommended.

- A can-opener technique may be performed with confidence in the majority of patients younger than age 10. The resilient anterior capsule contracts postoperatively, and the multiple can-opener leaflets often stretch into a perfect circle soon after surgery. The can-opener technique is helpful in cases of poor visualization and white cataract. Radial tearing is rare.

- Anterior capsulotomy can be performed with the automated vitrector, as popularized by Dr. ME Wilson.[23-23] There is no need to initiate a flap with the cystotome. The anterior capsule is directly engaged by the automated vitrector at a low cut rate, and the desired capsulotomy size is vitrected. A vitrector supported by a Venturi pump is helpful, since peristaltic pump systems are ineffective at cutting the anterior capsule.

- Radiofrequency thermal cautery capsulotomy is a new capsulotomy technique not yet in widespread use.[24] The Kloti radiofrequency diathermy handpiece is a platinum alloy-tipped probe that uses a high-frequency current (500 kHz) to incise the anterior capsule. The tip heats to about 160°C and cauterizes the capsule on contact. This technique may minimize capsulorrhexis complications, although the cauterized capsular edge has been noted to be more brittle and less elastic than in CCC or vitrectomized capsulotomies. This eliminates the risk of radial tears and produces a stable, accurately sized capsulotomy.

Hydrodissection

Hydrodissection is critical in the pediatric cataract, enhancing cortical clean-up and reducing severity of postoperative inflammation. In cases of posterior lenticonus, hydrodissection should be performed very gently since pre-existing posterior capsular dehiscence is often present.

Lens Aspiration

Automated irrigation and aspiration is usually sufficient for removal of the soft nucleus and cortex. Given the soft homogeneous lens material, thorough hydrodissection obviates the need for hydrodelineation. In cases of posterior capsular rupture, lens sheets glide and viscotamponades are often unnecessary because of the formed nature of pediatric vitreous. However, efflux of lens material into the vitreous chamber will require pars plana vitrectomy, ideally at the time of cataract extraction.

Some surgeons recommend using a permanent anterior chamber maintainer (ACM) throughout the case to maintain inflation of the soft eye and to provide more room to maneuver within the deeper anterior chamber.

Cortical Aspiration

If the irrigation and aspiration tip was used for nuclear/cortical removal, then cortical clean-up follows as a matter of course with the same instrument tip. The phacoemulsification probe should not be used for cortical clean-up to avoid unintentional capsular rupture.

Special Techniques: Posterior Capsulotomy

The reported incidence of posterior capsular opacification ranges from 33% to 100% in congenital cataracts. In children under the age of 6, primary posterior capsulotomy and limited anterior vitrectomy is standard to prevent exuberant posterior capsular fibrosis.[25-28] The posterior capsulotomy should be slightly smaller than the anterior capsulotomy to enhance IOL stability or facilitate future placement of a secondary IOL. Controversy surrounds whether an anterior vitrectomy is needed to prevent secondary membrane growth across the anterior vitreous face.

- Posterior capsulotomy is most commonly achieved with posterior vitrectorrhexis. The initial capsulotomy puncture can be carried out with a cystotome. The resultant flap is engaged with the vitrector, and the desired capsulotomy is then sculpted. Alternatively, the vitrector can be used to directly engage the posterior capsule.

- Posterior CCC may also be employed but increases surgical time and manipulation and may be associated with technical complications. Adequate viscoelastic agent must be used to counteract the anterior vector forces exerted by the ballooning vitreous, and precise control of the posterior capsular leaflet again requires capsular forceps. The vitrectomy probe can then be introduced into the eye to carry out the anterior vitrectomy. This technique risks leaving residual viscoelastic.

- If there is access to a ceiling-mounted YAG laser, posterior capsulotomy may be performed at the conclusion of surgery without specific need for anterior vitrectomy.[25]

IOL Implantation

Posterior in-the-bag lens implantation is the preferred IOL implantation technique. The capsular leaflets are separated using viscoelastic to create space for the IOL. If a foldable IOL is used, the lens is unfolded in the anterior chamber with the leading haptic in the bag and the trailing haptic outside the eye. The trailing haptic is then dunked or dialed into position as usual. Ciliary sulcus placement may be done if integrity of the capsular bag is in question. Both haptics must be placed in the same anatomic location to prevent decentration.

Howard Gimbel describes placing the IOL in the bag, reaching beneath the IOL to create a posterior CCC, then prolapsing the optic through the posterior opening.[26-28] This technique may lessen posterior capsular fibrosis by reducing contact between the IOL and the interior aspect of the capsular bag.

Wound Closure

A self-sealing wound is not reliable in pediatric cases, and wound suturing is imperative. It is nearly impossible to prevent children from rubbing their eyes, so the risk of trauma is greatly increased in this population.[6] Furthermore, the decreased scleral rigidity in the pediatric eye leads to a less stable wound. Therefore, watertight closure with multiple interrupted 8-0 Vicryl sutures is necessary. "No stitch" or "one stitch" surgery should not be performed. Wound prolapse should not occur if interrupted sutures are employed in the wound closure.[7]

Immediate Postoperative Medications

Routine subconjunctival injections of antibiotics and steroids are often employed at the conclusion of the case, although efficacy has yet to be proven in a clinical study.

Acetazolamide may be used if one suspects residual viscoelastic agent in the eye or if postoperative IOP spikes are anticipated and accurate IOP monitoring is not possible. However, postoperative acetazolamide in the nonglaucomatous patient is not routine, since children tolerate IOP increases better than adults.

RELEVANT POSTOPERATIVE ISSUES

Complications

1. Inflammatory response. Even in uneventful cases of pediatric cataract extraction, intense inflammation is a common postoperative complication, especially in cases with IOL implantation. Compliance with eye drops is essential.

2. IOP spikes. These are not uncommon and may be due to a variety of causes, including uveitis, angle closure, uveal effusion, and pre-existing open-angle glaucoma or angle abnormalities.[29] Treatment is tailored according to the etiology of the IOP spike; however, the greatest challenge may be in accurate monitoring of IOP. Exam under anesthesia (EUA), when necessary, may greatly facilitate appropriate therapy.

3. Postoperative retinal detachment is rare in the pediatric population, perhaps because of the robust vitality of the pediatric retinal pigment epithelium and formed vitreous. Suspected detachment should be referred to the appropriate specialist.

4. Postoperative endophthalmitis is uncommon and is managed with intravitreal antibiotics and possible vitrectomy with IOL removal.[30,31]

Postoperative Medications

1. Topical cycloplegics with cyclopentolate 0.5% bid in children younger than 6 months, or a stronger concentration in older children, minimizes formation of posterior synechiae.

2. Antibiotic/steroid combination drops are prudent to simplify the drop schedule and enhance compliance.

3. With intense inflammation, prednisolone acetate is required.

Follow-Up

1. Eye patches should be removed on postoperative day 1 and replaced with a clear plastic shield to encourage use of the eye as soon as possible in patients under 10, minimizing the risk of amblyopia. If amblyopia is suspected, commence patching of the contralateral eye at 1 week postoperatively.

2. Persistent attempts to accurately check eye pressure should be made. EUA should be considered in glaucoma suspects in whom accurate IOP cannot be obtained.

3. Dilate the pupil frequently in the initial postoperative period to prevent adhesions between the posterior iris and the anterior capsule.

4. Refract the patient as early as 2 weeks after surgery to identify any refractive surprises. Glasses or contact lenses may be fitted at approximately 4 weeks, when the wound is considered stable.

5. The frequency of surgical follow-up is dictated by success of the surgery, the healing response of the child, status of amblyopia, and the presence of glaucoma or other ocular defects.

When to Consider Alternative Procedures

1. Sensory strabismus or nystagmus are poor prognostic factors for postoperative vision, possibly influencing initial consideration of surgery.

2. Distorted globe dimensions such as microphthalmos and microcornea technically complicate surgery and adversely affect surgical success.

3. Concomitant ocular abnormalities such as glaucoma, retinal disease, optic nerve disease, PHPV, or ROP. These conditions portend poorer prognosis than cataract alone. Consider combined procedures if indicated. Consider avoiding surgery if the visual prognosis is poor.

4. Unilateral cataracts. These patients often achieve visual acuity of 20/100 or worse despite aggressive amblyopia therapy.[10] Consider avoiding surgery especially if concomitant diseases are severe.

5. History of uveitis. IOLs are contraindicated in patients with active uveitis. Leave patient aphakic.

6. Compromised visual-evoked response (VER) or ERG values. These studies provide gross assessment of visual prognosis. If visual prognosis is poor, consider canceling surgery.

Key Points

1. If the posterior segment cannot be visualized, a preoperative B-scan must be performed.

2. Rule out concomitant ocular and systemic conditions.

3. Maximize therapy of treatable conditions such as glaucoma.

4. Remove visually significant cataracts as soon as possible.

5. Refract eye within 2 to 3 weeks to identify refractive surprises.

6. Provide aggressive amblyopia treatment pre- and postoperatively.

7. Use deep general anesthesia with muscle paralysis.

8. Consider IOL placement in children older than 2 years of age. For children without primary IOL placement, preserve enough capsule to support a secondary IOL at a later date.

9. Avoid ACIOLs.

10. Perform a primary posterior capsulotomy wherever possible.

11. Suture the wound.

REFERENCES

1. Foster A, Gilbert C, Rahi J. Epidemiology of cataract in childhood: a global perspective. *J Cataract Refract Surg.* 1997;23(1):601-604.

2. Lambert SR, Drack AV. Infantile cataracts. *Surv Ophthalmol.* 1996;40(6):427-458.

3. Biglan AW. Pediatric patients. In: Lu LW, Fine IH, ed. *Phacoemulsification in Difficult and Challenging Cases.* New York: Thieme; 1999:129-143.

4. Lambert SR. Lens. In: Taylor D, ed. *Paediatric Ophthalmology.* London: Blackwell Science Ltd; 1997: 445-476.

5. Arkin M, Azar D, Fraioli A. Infantile cataracts. *Int Ophthalmol Clin.* 1992;32(1):107-120.

6. Simons BD, Siatkowski RM, Schiffman JC, et al. Surgical technique, visual outcome, and complications of pediatric intraocular lens implantation. *J Pediatr Ophthalmol Strabismus.* 1999;36(3):118-124.

7. Sharma N, Pushker N, Dada T, et al. Complications of pediatric cataract surgery and intraocular lens implantation. *J Cataract Refract Surg.* 1999;25(12):1585-1588.

8. Zwaan J, Mullaney PB, Awad A, et al. Pediatric intraocular lens implantation. Surgical results and complications in more than 300 patients. *Ophthalmology.* 1998;105(1):112-118.

9. Basti S, Aasuri MK, Reddy MK, et al. Heparin-surface-modified intraocular lenses in pediatric cataract surgery: prospective randomized study. *J Cataract Refract Surg.* 1999;25(6):782-787.

10. Greenwald MJ, Glaser SR. Visual outcomes after surgery for unilateral cataract in children more than two years old: posterior chamber intraocular lens implantation versus contact lens correction of aphakia. *J AAPOS.* 1998;2(3):168-176.

11. Asrani S, Freedman S, Hasselblad V, et al. Does primary intraocular lens implantation prevent "aphakic" glaucoma in children? *Journal of AAPOS.* 2000;4:33-39.

12. Enyedi LB, Peterseim MW, Freedman SF, et al. Refractive changes after pediatric intraocular lens implantation. *Am J Ophthalmol.* 1998;126:772-781.

13. Griener ED, Dahan E, Lambert SR. Effect of age at time of cataract surgery on subsequent axial length growth in infant eyes. *J Cataract Refract Surg.* 1999;25:1209-1213.

14. Hutchinson AK, Drews-Botsch C, Lambert SR. Myopic shift after intraocular lens implantation during childhood. *Ophthalmology.* 1997;104:1752-1757.

15. Hutchinson AK, Wilson ME, Saunders RA. Outcomes and ocular growth rates after intraocular lens implantation in the first 2 years of life. *J Cataract Refract Surg.* 1998;24:846-852.

16. McClatchey SK, Parks MM. Theoretic refractive changes after lens implantation in childhood. *Ophthalmology.* 1997;104:1744-1751.

17. McClatchey SK, Parks MM. Myopic shift after cataract removal in childhood. *J Pediatr Ophthalmol Strabismus.* 1997;34:88-95.

18. McClatchey SK, Dahan E, Males E, et al. A comparison of the rate of refractive growth in pediatric aphakic and pseudophakic eyes. *Ophthalmology.* 2000;107:118-122.

19. Dahan E, Drusedau MU. Choice of lens and dioptric power in pediatric pseudophakia. *J Cataract Refract Surg.* 1997;23:618-623.

20. McClatchey SK. Intraocular lens calculator for childhood cataract. *J Cataract Refract Surg.* 1998;24(8):1125-1129.

21. Andreo LK, Wilson ME, Saunders RA. Predictive value of regression and theoretical IOL formulas in pediatric intraocular lens implantation. *J Pediatr Ophthalmol Strabismus.* 1997;34:240-243.

22. Wilson ME. Anterior capsule management for pediatric intraocular lens implantation. *J Pediatr Ophthalmol Strabismus.* 1999;36(6):314-319.

23. Andreo LK, Wilson ME, Apple DJ. Elastic properties and scanning electron microscopic appearance of manual continuous curvilinear capsulorrhexis and vitrectorrhexis in an animal model of pediatric cataract. *J Cataract Refract Surg.* 1999;25(4):534-539.

24. Comer RM, Abdulla N, O'Keefe M. Radiofrequency diathermy capsulorrhexis of the anterior and posterior capsules in pediatric cataract surgery: preliminary results. *J Cataract Refract Surg.* 1997;23(1):641-644.

25. Fenton S, O'Keefe M. Primary posterior capsulorrhexis without anterior vitrectomy in pediatric cataract surgery: longer-term outcome. *J Cataract Refract Surg.* 1999;25(6):763-767.

26. Gimbel HV, DeBroff BM. Posterior capsulorrhexis with optic capture: maintaining a clear visual axis after pediatric cataract surgery. *J Cataract Refract Surg.* 1994;20:658-664.

27. Gimbel HV. Posterior capsulorrhexis with optic capture in pediatric cataract and intraocular lens surgery. *Ophthalmology.* 1996;103:1871-1875.

28. Gimbel HV. Posterior continuous curvilinear capsulorrhexis and optic capture of the intraocular lens to prevent secondary opacification in pediatric cataract surgery. *J Cataract Refract Surg.* 1997;23:652-626.

29. Egbert JE, Wright MM, Dahlhauser KF, et al. A prospective study of ocular hypertension and glaucoma after pediatric cataract surgery. *Ophthalmology.* 1995;102(7):1098-1101.

30. Wheeler DT, Stager DR, Weakley DR Jr. Endophthalmitis following pediatric intraocular surgery for congenital cataracts and congenital glaucoma. *J Pediatr Ophthalmol Strabismus.* 1992;29(3):139-141.

31. Good WV, Hing S, Irvine AR, et al. Postoperative endophthalmitis in children following cataract surgery. *J Pediatr Ophthalmol Strabismus.* 1990;27(6):283-285.

15

INTRAOCULAR LENS CALCULATIONS AFTER REFRACTIVE SURGERY

Roberto Pineda II, MD

RELEVANT PREOPERATIVE ISSUES

Clinical Setting

With an estimated 1.7 million cases performed in 2000, LASIK has entered the mainstream. LASIK has come to dominate refractive surgery, overtaking previous procedures such as radial keratotomy (RK) and photorefractive keratectomy (PRK). As baby boomers and older patients embrace refractive surgery, we will see a growing number of refractive surgery patients who present with visually significant cataracts.

Increased public awareness about cataract surgery, with greater emphasis on expected visual outcomes, has heightened the importance of accuracy in IOL power calculations. Because corneal refractive surgery changes the shape of the cornea, it also affects the actual keratometric measurements and makes the usually uncomplicated IOL calculation similar to sailing without a compass.

Although surgical techniques for phacoemulsification and IOL implantation are not generally felt to be different in patients who have had refractive surgery, IOL power calculations are unquestionably more complex in these patients. Standard IOL power formulas using routine keratometry (average K-readings) yield significant undercorrections with postoperative hyperopic endpoints (hyperopic surprise) in patients who have undergone RK, PRK, or LASIK.[1,2] Thus, determining the appropriate IOL power for these patients challenges many phacoemulsification surgeons.

This chapter reviews the fundamentals of IOL power calculations and discusses sources of inaccuracy using our current methodology and technology. Several methods for minimizing IOL power calculation errors will be presented.

IOL Power Formulas

Axial length measurements and keratometry readings form the cornerstone of accurate IOL power selection. Axial length measurements are often thought to be the greatest source of error; in fact, inaccurate keratometric measurements contribute more to IOL power miscalculations in patients who have undergone corneal refractive surgery.

To help understand how keratometry affects IOL power, it helps to review the original SRK formula. This formula is as follows:

$$P = A - 2.5L - 0.9K$$

> P = IOL power for emmetropia (D); A = constant specific to IOL (no units); L = axial length (mm); K = average keratometric measurement (D)

As one can see, an overestimated or higher keratometry reading will result in a lower estimation of IOL power. Underpowering the IOL causes a hyperopic surprise. For example, a myope after refractive surgery may have measured average keratometry readings of 44.00, but a true central corneal power of 42.00. Using standard IOL power calculations, this person would experience a hyperopic surprise after cataract surgery. The converse is true for a hyperopic patient, who will have underestimated keratometry readings and an overpowered IOL, resulting in a myopic surprise.

While today the SRK formula is obsolete and third-generation IOL power formulas have become the standard of care, all IOL calculation formulas to date rely on keratometry readings. Some of the most commonly used include:

1. 1988: Holladay I
2. 1990: SRK/T
3. 1992: Hoffer Q
4. 1996: Holladay II

Listed in Appendix A are the IOL power formula recommendations based on axial lengths.

Keratometry Determination

Before refractive surgery, the cornea is aspheric with a generally spherical central cornea and slightly flatter periphery. This is referred to as a prolate configuration. However, after myopic keratorefractive surgery, this profile is reversed, and the central cornea is flattened while the peripheral cornea steepens. This is called an oblate configuration. The opposite is true for hyperopic refractive corneal surgery when the cornea assumes an even more prolate configuration.[3]

Accurate keratometry measurements are critical to achieving a satisfactory refractive result after cataract surgery. Unfortunately, there is currently no good method for measuring keratometry after corneal refractive surgery. We are limited by the available technology. Current methods for measuring keratometric diopters include manual keratometry, automated keratometry, and corneal videokeratography (corneal topography). All of these techniques measure points outside the central cornea and therefore record an inaccurate central corneal power (higher in myopes and lower in hyperopes). While hyperopes have a myopic surprise after cataract surgery and myopes have a hyperopic surprise, the errors in myopes tend to be greater.

Manual keratometry is thought to be the least accurate method for determining keratometric D after keratorefractive surgery because only four opposing points (separated by about 3.2 mm) are measured in the paracentral cornea. Automated keratometry may be better than manual keratometry since it measures an area closer to the central cornea (about 2.6 mm).

Corneal topography is generally thought to yield the best approximation of central corneal power since it can sample thousands of points on the cornea, including many within the central 3 mm. Compared with keratometry, corneal topography may also provide greater accuracy in evaluating corneal power when there is irregular astigmatism. Additionally, several of the corneal topography units offer central corneal diagnostic parameters such as the "average central power" and the "effective refractive power." These parameters may have added value in determining actual central corneal power. It is recommended that several different measurements be obtained for comparison.

Etiologies of keratometric error differ for RK versus PRK/LASIK and should be considered separately.[4] PRK/LASIK will be discussed first. In these cases, the major sources of error are inaccurate anterior curvature measurements and changes in the corneal index of refraction. Moreover, the magnitude of error in the keratometric readings and IOL power selection has been correlated with the depth of the ablation.

Inaccurate anterior corneal measurements in PRK/LASIK occur due to flattening or steepening of the cornea. With flattening, the diameter of the spherical corneal circle that is measured increases, and the keratometry measurement points become farther apart and farther away from the central cornea. Conversely, steepening the cornea moves the points closer together. Both changes alter the keratometric measurements such that they reflect the central corneal power less accurately.

In PRK/LASIK, the index of refraction is affected as well. This effect is due to alterations in the ratio of anterior to posterior curvature, as well to the decrease in central corneal thickness.[5] For example, with myopic PRK/LASIK, tissue removal from the anterior corneal surface leads to anterior corneal flattening, while the posterior cornea remains relatively unchanged. Thus, the ratio of anterior to posterior curvature increases, and the central corneal thickness decreases. However, since standard keratometry only measures the anterior surface of the cornea (assuming a constant refractive index of the cornea), it cannot detect changes in central corneal thickness or anterior/posterior curvature ratios. Standard methods of keratometry overestimate the central corneal power of post-PRK/LASIK corneas in myopes and underestimate its power in hyperopes.

In contrast, in radial keratometry, the two main reasons for inaccurate keratometric D readings include irregular central corneal astigmatism and misreading of the anterior corneal curvature. Irregular central astigmatism can be caused by uneven incisions and/or asymmetric healing of the cornea. Misreading of the anterior corneal curvature in RK occurs because the central RK incisions create a paracentral "knee" in the cornea curvature; the keratometric measurements fall on the steep part of the knee, thereby overestimating the central corneal power. This effect is further amplified by corneal flattening that actually moves the keratometry readings farther from the central cornea, magnifying the error in keratometric measurements. This error increases with a greater number of RK incisions and smaller optical zones.

Unlike PRK/LASIK, changes in the corneal index of refraction are not a factor. The deep radial incisions used to correct myopia in RK indirectly cause flattening of the central cornea through midperipheral bulging. Since no tissue is removed in this technique, the anterior and posterior corneal surfaces respond in a similar fashion, and the index of refraction is unchanged.

STRATEGIES TO MAXIMIZE OUTCOMES

1. Obtain consent from the patient. Be sure to discuss with the patient the difficulty in calculating the lens implant power and the need for possible IOL exchange after surgery. Also reinforce that any optical aberrations after the previous refractive procedure will not be "fixed" by cataract surgery. This discussion is important so that both the physician and the patient will have realistic expectations after the cataract surgery. Such discussion will also lessen the risk that the patient will blame the surgeon for refractive surgery-related symptoms after cataract extraction.

2. For patients with fluctuating vision after refractive surgery (especially RK), consider measuring the keratometric D both in the morning and in the afternoon. Factor these fluctuations into the equation such that the patient is plano in the morning and myopic in the afternoon. This strategy avoids periods of hyperopia, which often make patients very unhappy.

3. In patients who have had RK, perform an endothelial cell count and pachymetry preoperatively since endothelial cell loss has been reported in these patients. For patients with borderline or low readings, it may be prudent to defer surgery until the cataract becomes very problematic for the patient due to the risk of corneal decompensation and bullous keratopathy.

Methods for Calculating Central Corneal Power after Refractive Surgery

Until better technology is developed for measuring true central corneal power, surgeons must rely on techniques that provide the best possible estimates. Currently, two methods have been described for approximating the actual central corneal power. These are the clinical history method and the hard contact lens method.[6,7]

1. The clinical history method requires knowledge of three parameters:

   • Keratometry readings prior to refractive surgery
   • Preoperative refractive surgery refraction (use spherical equivalent)
   • Postoperative refraction 6 weeks to 6 months after refractive surgery

   To perform this calculation, use the patient's preoperative "average K's." Let's say the K's are 45.50 D/46.50 D at 90 preoperatively. This means that the average K is 46 D. Next, if we know that the preoperative spherical equivalent (SE) was -4.50 D and the postoperative SE was +0.50 D, we can calculate that a 5.00 D hyperopic change occurred (-4.50 to +0.50). By subtracting the change in diopters from the preoperative average K, the new central corneal power can be determined (46 – 5 = 41 D). Adjusting for vertex distance back to the corneal plane is not necessary, since even for high myopes the error is minor and in the myopic direction.

   New central corneal power = 46 D (preoperative average K) – 5 D (net change in refraction) = 41 D

The major problem with using this method is that often the necessary preoperative measurements are not available, so the calculations cannot be performed. A second problem can be instability of the postoperative refraction, since cataracts often cause myopic shift. Using a recent refraction (which reflects this myopic shift) to calculate the net refractive change after refractive surgery will result in miscalculation with a hyperopic endpoint. For example, if a patient was -8.00 D before refractive surgery and plano afterward, then underwent a myopic shift of -2.00 D due to the cataract, the apparent net refractive change would be -6.00 D rather than the actual -8.00 D. This miscalculation would cause a 2 D hyperopic error.

2. The hard contact lens method requires less information:

- No clinical history is needed.
- Vision must be correctable to 20/80 or better.
- A plano hard contact lens (HCL) of known base curve (eg, 40 D) is needed. The base curve of the HCL should be within 3 D of the anticipated central corneal power to achieve the most accurate result.
- First, refract the patient without the HCL and record the SE.
- Then, refract the patient with the HCL.
- Calculate the net difference between the two refractions (with and without the HCL).
- Add or subtract the difference to the dioptric power (base curve) of the HCL.

For instance, if a patient was +0.25 D without a HCL and -1.75 D with a 40 D HCL in place, then the net refractive change is -2.00 D. The patient's central corneal power reading can be calculated as follows:

Central corneal power = 40 D (HCL) – 2.00 D (net refractive change with HCL) – 38 D

The main disadvantage with this technique is that it requires vision to be correctable to 20/80 before cataract surgery. This method is best combined with other methods. When combining methods for myopes, one should always choose the flattest central corneal power predicted to avoid hyperopic surprises.

For patients who do not have clinical information prior to refractive surgery and whose vision is worse than 20/80, use the effective refractive power (ERP) parameter on the Holladay diagnostic summary, or the average central power (ACP) on the TSM-1 unit.

RELEVANT POSTOPERATIVE ISSUES

Complications

1. Unexpected refractive error. Review preoperative data and consider IOL exchange once the refraction has stabilized.
2. Patients who have had RK may experience a significant hyperopic shift immediately after cataract surgery due to corneal edema, similar to that experienced after their refractive surgery. Additional corneal flattening may occur. Do not attempt an IOL exchange until 1 to 3 months after surgery when the refraction has stabilized since this hyperopic shift often improves.[1]

3. In RK patients, diurnal fluctuations in vision are not uncommon after cataract surgery. By accounting for this possibility preoperatively, hyperopic periods can be avoided.

WHEN TO CONSIDER ALTERNATIVE PROCEDURES

Patients who have had RK may be at risk for bullous keratopathy after cataract surgery. Consider delaying surgery if endothelial cell count and pachymetry are abnormal. If the patient has advanced cataracts with corneal changes, consider combined corneal transplant and cataract surgery.

KEY POINTS

1. Extensively discuss risks and benefits with the patient so that realistic expectations are achieved.

2. Corneal topography should be performed in all patients to evaluate asphericity and irregular astigmatism.

3. Use the flattest K-readings for myopes.

4. Use the steepest K-readings for hyperopes.

5. For myopes, use multiple third-generation formulas for the IOL power calculation and choose the highest calculated power implant. The opposite is true for hyperopes.

6. The clinical history method should be applied whenever possible for myopes or hyperopes.

7. Obtain a set of plano HCLs of different base curves (ie, 35 D, 40 D, and 45 D) in order to accurately use the HCL method.

REFERENCES

1. Koch DD, Liu JF, Hyde LL, et al. Refractive complications of cataract surgery after radial keratotomy. Am J Ophthalmol. 1989;108:676-682.

2. Lyle WA, Jin GJC. Intraocular lens power prediction in patients who undergo cataract surgery following previous radial keratotomy. Arch Ophthalmol. 1997:115;457-461.

3. Holladay JT. Cataract surgery in patients with previous keratorefractive surgery (RK, PRK, and LASIK). Ophthalmic Pract. 1997:15:238-244.

4. Seitz B, Langenbucher A. Intraocular lens calculations status after corneal refractive surgery. Curr Opin Ophthalmol. 2000;11(1):35-46.

5. Mandell RB. Corneal power correction factor for photorefractive keratectomy. J Refract Corneal Surg. 1994;10:125-128.

6. Seitz B, Langenbucher A, Nguyen NX, et al. Underestimation of intraocular lens power for cataract surgery after myopic photorefractive keratectomy. Ophthalmology. 1999;106:693-702.

7. Hoffer KJ. Intraocular lens power calculation for eyes after refractive keratotomy. J Refract Surg. 1995;11:490-493.

A

RECOMMENDED INTRAOCULAR LENS POWER FORMULAS BASED ON AXIAL LENGTH

FORMULA	AXIAL LENGTH	% OF EYES IN POPULATION
Hoffer-Q	<22 mm	8%
Holladay II	<22 mm	8%
Holladay I	24.5 to 26.0 mm	15%
SRK-T	>26 mm	5%
Average	22.0 to 24.5 mm	72%

Keratometry readings and axial length are the cornerstones of IOL formulas. Although the accuracy of today's third generation IOL power calculation formulas have improved our ability to predict the patient's final refraction, no IOL formula works well at all axial lengths. Moreover, it has been shown that certain IOL formulas perform better, particularly at extreme axial lengths. Listed above are four commonly used modern IOL formulas. Two of these formulas, the Hoffer-Q and the Holladay II, have been shown to be good predictors of final target refraction for eyes with short axial lengths (>22 mm). In contrast, eyes with medium to long axial lengths (24 to 26 mm), achieve better results with the Holladay I formula. Finally, for long axial lengths (>26 mm), the SRK/T formula appears to be the most accurate. For axial lengths between 22.0 and 24.5 mm, the average of three formulas (Hoffer-Q, Holladay I, and SRK/T) is used to determine the IOL power. The Holladay II is the newest IOL formula that uses additional parameters, such as corneal diameter and axial length, when determining the IOL power. This formula is not yet published.

REFERENCE

1. Hoffer KJ. Clinical results using the Holladay II intraocular lens power formula. *J Cataract Refract Surg*. 2000;26(8):1233-1237.

B

LIMBAL RELAXING INCISION NOMOGRAM
(600-MICRON DEPTH)[1,2]

Limbal relaxing incisions (LRIs) (Figure B-1) are a convenient, easy technique for the correction of keratometric (corneal) astigmatism. Approximately 25% of patients undergoing cataract surgery have ≥ 1.25 D of keratometric astigmatism. LRIs can be performed at the start or finish of surgery, or performed as a secondary procedure. This procedure is generally more effective for with-the-rule astigmatism (in the vertical meridian) and should be based on corneal topography and keratometry.

Procedure

1. Preoperatively, keratometry and corneal topography should be performed. LRIs should be based on corneal astigmatism and not the patient's preoperative refraction since lenticular astigmatism is not a consideration. Preoperative corneal pachymetry is not necessary since the normal peripheral cornea measures 800 to 1000 microns. Patients with peripheral corneal pathology should not have LRI's.

2. Intraoperatively, after the eye has been prepped and draped for surgery, a degree gauge is used to mark the steep axis and/or fixate the globe (Figure B-2).

3. Use inked calipers to mark the chord length (6 mm, 8 mm, or 10 mm) based on the above modified Gills nomogram (see Figure B-1).

4. Set the diamond blade for 600 microns or use a preset 600-micron sapphire or steel blade. Firmly place the blade at the start of the incision, pull slowly through the tissue observing the blade closely (corneal perforation is a rare occurrence).

5. Incisions may be enhanced intraoperatively or postoperatively if necessary.

6. Perform routine clear corneal or scleral tunnel phacoemulsification. Alternatively, the order can be changed and the LRIs can be performed at the end of the surgery. This is not our preference due to wound leak.

Figure B-1. Limbal relaxing incisions.

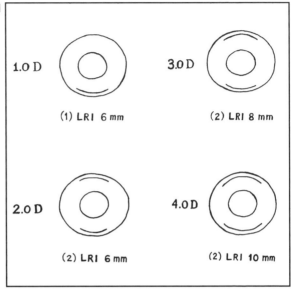

Figure B-2. Intraoperatively, after the eye has been prepped and draped for surgery, a degree gauge is used to mark the steep axis and/or fixate the globe.

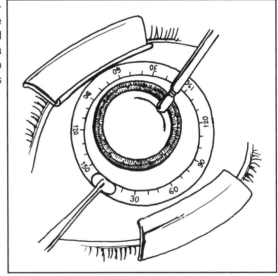

REFERENCES

1. Budak K, Friedman NJ, Koch DD. Limbal relaxing incisions with cataract surgery. *J Cataract Refract Surg.* 1998:24(4):503-508.
2. Muller-Jensen K, Fischer P, Siepe U. Limbal relaxing incisions to correct astigmatism in clear corneal cataract surgery. *J Refract Corneal Surg.* 1999;15(5):586-589.

C

ALGORITHM FOR PSEUDOPHAKIC CYSTOID MACULAR EDEMA[1-3]

After posterior capsular opacification, cystoid macular edema (CME) is the most common cause of visual loss related to cataract surgery. This condition may persist for as long as 1 year or more after surgery, occasionally leading to permanent reduction in vision. Decreased contrast sensitivity is also a frequent finding.

We present this algorithm on the next page for managing CME based on our own experience and review of the literature. Predisposing conditions for CME include diabetes, uveitis, planned sutured PCIOL, and history of CME in the other eye. Surgical high-risk conditions where violation of the posterior capsule is more likely and the CME risk is greater include posterior polar cataract, pseudoexfoliation (PXF), hard and dense nuclei, white cataracts, and traumatic cataracts.

NOTES REGARDING THE FOLLOWING DIAGRAMS

1. Topical NSAIDs may be toxic to the corneal epithelium.

2. Polishing the lens capsule removes epithelial cells. These cells are a source of prostaglandin production, and may contribute to CME.

3. Our subtenon's injection is usually dosed at 20 to 40 mg of triamcinalone.

4. Response to CME treatment is determined by either improvement in visual acuity or patients' subjective complaints.

5. Acetazolamide is not recommended for patients with sulfa allergies or kidney disease.

6. Review gastrointestinal status and history of gastric ulcers with patients before starting oral NSAIDs or steroids.

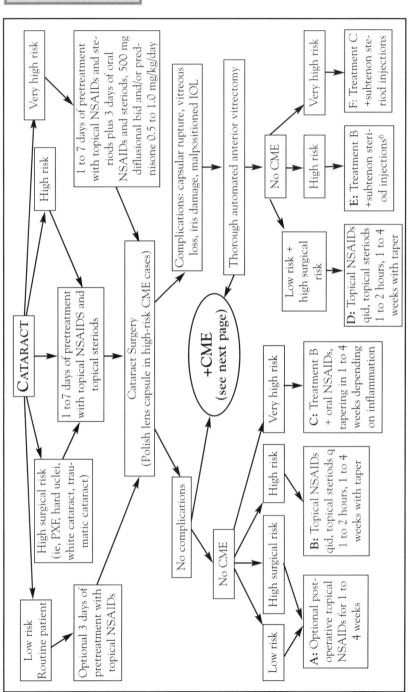

Flow Diagram 1.

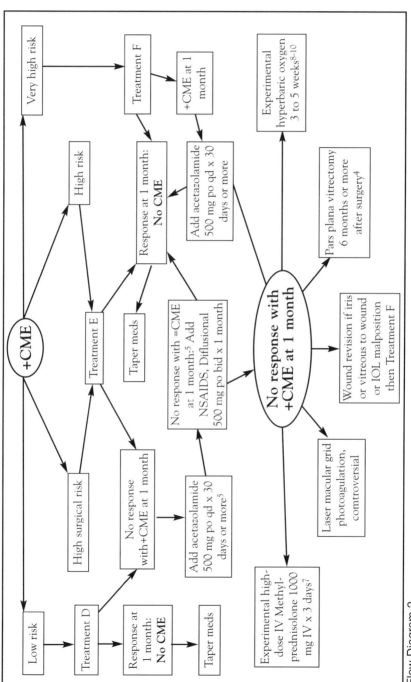

Flow Diagram 2.

REFERENCES

1. Rossetti L, Chaidhuri J, Dickersin K. Medical prophylaxis and treatment of cystoid macular edema after cataract surgery. *Ophthalmology*. 1998;105:397-405.

2. Rossetti L, Autelitano A. Cystoid macular edema following cataract surgery. *Curr Opin Ophthalmol*. 2000;11(1):65-72.

3. Flach AJ. The incidence, pathogenesis and treatment of cystoid macular edema following cataract surgery. *Trans Am Ophthalmol Soc*. 1998;96:557-634.

4. Pendergast SD, Margherio RR, Williams GA, et al. Vitrectomy for chronic pseudophakic cystoid macular edema. *Am J Ophthalmol*. 1999;128(3):317-323.

5. Wolfensberger TJ. The role of carbonic anhydrase inhibitors in the management of macular edema. *Doc Ophthalmol*. 1999;97(3-4):387-397.

6. Thach AB, Dugel PU, Flindall RJ, et al. A comparison of retrobulbar versus sub-Tenon's corticosteroid therapy for cystoid macular edema refractory to topical medications. *Ophthalmology* 1997;104(12):2003-2008.

7. Abe T, Hayasaka S, Nagaki Y, et al. Pseudophakic cystoid macular edema treated with high-dose intravenous methylprednisolone. *J Cataract Refract Surg*. 1999;25(9):1286-1288.

8. Pfoff DS, Thom SR. Preliminary report on the effect of hyperbaric oxygen on cystoid macular edema. *J Cataract Refract Surg*. 1987;13(2):136-140.

9. Suttorp-Schulten MSA, Van Der Kley AJ, Riemslag FCC. Long-term effect of repeated hyperbaric oxygen therapy on visual acuity in inflammatory cystoid macular oedema. *Br J Ophthalmol*. 1997;81:329.

10. Miyake Y, Awaya S, Takahashi H, et al. Hyperbaric oxygen and acetazolamide improve visual acuity in patients with cystoid macular edema by different mechanisms. *Arch Ophthalmol*. 1993;111:1605-1606.

LEVELS OF DIABETIC RETINOPATHY: ETDRS CLASSIFICATION AND CRITERIA FOR Rx[1,2]

NPDR	CHARACTERISTICS
Mild NPDR	• At least one microaneurysm • Characteristics not met for more severe DR
Moderate NPDR	• Hemorrhages and/or microaneurysms (H/ma) of moderate degree (ie, > standard ETDRS photograph 2A) • Soft exudates (cotton wool spots), venous beading, or intraretinal microvascular abnormalities (IRMA) definitely present • Characteristics not met for more severe NPDR

Severe NPDR	• One of the following:
	  • H/Ma > standard ETDRS photograph 2A in four retinal quadrants.
	  • Venous beading in two retinal quadrants > standard ETDRS photo 6B
	  • IRMA in 1 retinal quadrant > standard ETDRS photo 8A
	• Characteristics not met for more severe DR

Very severe NPDR	• Two or more lesions of severe NPDR • No frank neovascularizations

PROLIFERATIVE DIABETIC RETINOPATHY (PDR)	CHARACTERISTICS
Early PDR	• New vessels definitely present • Characteristics not met for more severe DR

High risk PDR	• One of more of the following:
	  • Neovascularization on the disc (NVD) $\geq$ one-fourth to one-third disc area (ie, NVD $\geq$ standard ETDRS photo 10A)
	  • Any NVD + vitreous or preretinal hemorrhage
	  • Neovascularization elsewhere on the retina (NVE) $\geq$ one-half disc area + vitreous or preretinal hemorrhage

CLINICALLY SIGNIFICANT MACULAR EDEMA

Any one of the following lesions:

• Retinal thickening at or within 500 microns (one-third disc diameter) from the center of the macula.

• Hard exudates at or within 500 microns from the center of the macula with thickening of the adjacent retina.

• A zone or zones of retinal thickening $\geq$ one disc area in size, any portion of which is $\leq$ 1 disc diameter from the center of the macula.

REFERENCES

1. The Early Treatment Diabetic Retinopathy Study Research Group. Fundus photographic risk factors for progression of diabetic retinopathy: ETDRS report number 12. *Ophthalmology*. 1991;98:823-833.

2. The Early Treatment Diabetic Retinopathy Study Research Group. Grading diabetic retinopathy from stereoscopic color fundus photographs—an extension of the modified Airlie House classification: ETDRS report number 10. *Ophthalmology*. 1991;98:786-986.

APPENDIX

VISCOELASTIC DIRECTORY

Viscoelastics play an important role in anterior segment surgery, particularly in cataract surgery. This directory is designed to increase your basic understanding of their properties and aid in selecting the most appropriate viscoelastic for your complicated cataract procedures.

Cohesive viscoelastics maintain the anterior chamber and facilitate IOL implantation. Their main characteristic is that they stick to themselves and are easily aspirated all at once.

Dispersive viscoelastics are much better at coating surfaces (eg, endothelium) but are much more difficult to remove all at once, as they tend to break off in pieces.

See the directory on the next page.

Product Name	Components	Molecular Weight/ Viscosity	Shear Rate Centipose (cps)	Characteristics
Akorn Ophthalmics (Lincolnshire, Ill)				
Biolon	1% sodium hyaluronate 10 mg/ml	3 million daltons	215 K VO (cps)	Dispersive
Alcon Laboratories (Fort Worth, Tex)				
Viscoat	3% sodium hyaluronate/ 4% chondroitin sulfate	600,000 daltons/ 40,000 cps	sec-2	Dispersive
Provisc	1% sodium hyaluronate	2.4 million daltons/ 39,000 cps	sec-2	Cohesive
DuoVisc	1 syringe of Viscoat 1 syringe of Provisc			Dispersive/ Cohesive
Cellugel	Hydroxypropylmethylcellulose 2%	300,000 daltons/40,000 cps	20,000-	Dispersive
Allergan (Irvine, Calif)				
AMO Vitrax	3% sodium hyaluronate 30 mg/ml	500,000 daltons/40,000 cps	40,000 cps	Cohesive
Biolon	1% sodium hyaluronate 10 mg/ml	3 million daltons	215 K VO (cps)	Dispersive
Bausch & Lomb Surgical (St Louis, Mo)				
Amvisc	Sodium hyaluronate 12 mg/ml (1.2%)	2 million daltons/40,000 cs	2 sec-1	Cohesive
Amvisc Plus	Sodium hyaluronate 16 mg/ml (1.6%)	1.5 million daltons/55,000 cs	2 sec-1	Cohesive
Ocucoat	Hydroxypropylmethylcellulose 2%	80,000 daltons/8000 cps	2 sec-1	Dispersive
Pharmacia & Upjohn (Monrovia, Calif)				
Healon GV	Sodium hyaluronate 14 mg/ml	5 million daltons/ 2 million cps at zero shear	2 million	Cohesive
Healon	Sodium hyaluronate 10 mg/ml	4 million daltons/ 200,000 cps at zero shear	200,000	Cohesive

INDEX

BUILD *Your Library*

This book and many others on numerous different topics are available from SLACK Incorporated. For further information or a copy of our latest catalog, contact us at:

Professional Book Division
SLACK Incorporated
6900 Grove Road
Thorofare, NJ 08086 USA
Telephone: 1-856-848-1000
1-800-257-8290
Fax: 1-856-853-5991
E-mail: orders@slackinc.com
www.slackbooks.com

We accept most major credit cards and checks or money orders in US dollars drawn on a US bank. Most orders are shipped within 72 hours.

Contact us for information on recent releases, forthcoming titles, and bestsellers. If you have a comment about this title or see a need for a new book, direct your correspondence to the Editorial Director at the above address.

Thank you for your interest and we hope you found this work beneficial.